NEURO-LOGIC PROBLEMS

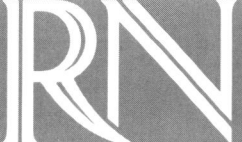

NURSING ASSESSMENT SERIES
DIANA I. BUBB, R.N., M.S.N.

Series Editor
Margaret Van Meter, R.N.
Clinical Editor, RN Magazine

MEDICAL ECONOMICS BOOKS
Oradell, New Jersey 07649

Library of Congress Cataloging in Publication Data

Bubb, Diana I.
  Neurologic problems.

  (RN nursing assessment series; 3)
  Includes index.
  1. Neurological nursing — Addresses, essays,
lectures. I. Title. II. Series: RN nursing assessment
series; v. 3. [DNLM: 1. Nervous system diseases — Nursing.
WY 100 R627 v. 3]
RC350.5.B83   1983   616.8   83-8228
ISBN 0-87489-287-2

Cover design by Jerry Wilke

ISBN 0-87489-287-2

Medical Economics Company Inc.
Oradell, New Jersey 07649

Printed in the United States of America

Copyright © 1984 by Medical Economics Company Inc., Oradell, NJ 07649. All rights reserved. None of the content of this publication may be reproduced, stored in a retrieval system, or transmitted in any form or by any means (electronic, mechanical, photocopying, recording, or otherwise) without the prior written permission of the publisher.

CONTENTS

Publisher's Notes	iv
1. Anatomy and Physiology of the Nervous System	1
2. The Neurologic History	27
3. Assessment of the Neurologic Patient	39
4. Alterations in Consciousness and Increased Intracranial Pressure	63
5. Nursing Management of the Neurologic Patient	77
6. Seizures	95
7. Cerebrovascular Diseases	109
8. Trauma to the Central Nervous System	127
9. Tumors of the Central Nervous System	143
10. Degenerative Diseases	159
11. Neuromuscular Diseases	177
12. Diagnostic Procedures	191
Appendix – Drugs Used for Neurologic Problems	208
Glossary	212
Additional Test Questions	215
Selected Readings	225
Index	230

PUBLISHER'S NOTES

Physical assessment is an integral part of the nursing process. Sharpening assessment skills, therefore, is bound to add logic and reason to planning, intervention, and evaluation. This volume in the *RN Nursing Assessment Series* focuses on assessment of neurologic function. It provides norms against which to compare pathologic findings.

For easy access, an outline format combined with a clear, concise test — an organizational scheme that has proven popular with nurses — was adopted. The illustrations, both halftone and line art, were selected specifically to add to the book's clarity and utility. Finally, the presentation of learning objectives and the inclusion of chapter quizzes, additional test questions, and a glossary make this book a learning/teaching tool.

Diana I. Bubb, R.N., M.S.N., is adjunct clinical assistant professor of nursing at Widener University School of Nursing in Chester, Pennsylvania. She has also taught neurologic/neurosurgical nursing in a diploma nursing program, as a staff development instructor, and in nursing continuing education programs, and has published articles in this field in *RN Magazine*. Margaret Van Meter, R.N., the series editor, is *RN Magazine*'s clinical editor for development and also serves as a private nurse consultant.

CHAPTER 1

Anatomy and Physiology of the Nervous System

OBJECTIVES

After completing this chapter, you will be able to:

1. Identify the cells of the nervous system, their components and function
2. Describe conduction of nerve impulses
3. Identify the structures of the central nervous system and their function
4. Describe the cerebral blood circulation
5. Describe cerebrospinal fluid production and circulation
6. Identify the cranial nerves and their functions
7. Discuss the components and function of the spinal nerves
8. Describe the divisions of the autonomic nervous system and their functions.

A. Introduction

Many nurses feel discouraged at the outset when studying the nervous system because it is complex, and because much has yet to be learned about its functioning. To provide optimal care for patients with neurologic dysfunction, however, it's vital that you understand the system's anatomy and physiology. Some concentration and study on your part should enable you to do so with relative ease. In fact, as you begin to apply your knowledge to direct patient care, you'll probably find the subject engrossing. This book is intended to help you reach that goal.

B. Cells of the nervous system

The two types of cells found in the nervous system are neuroglia cells and neurons.

1. Neuroglia cells

Neuroglia cells provide nourishment, protection, and structural support for neurons. There are four types of neuroglia cells:

a. Astrocytes. These cells contribute to neuronal nutrition, store information, maintain neuronal electrical potential, and help support the blood-brain barrier that surrounds the capillaries of the central nervous system (CNS).

b. Oligodendroglia. These cells form the myelin sheath around axons within the central nervous system.

c. Microglia. Microglia act as scavengers to remove microbes and cellular debris from the CNS, in a process called phagocytosis.

d. Ependymal cells. These cells line the ventricular system, the choroid plexi, and the central canal of the spinal cord.

2. Neurons

Neurons possess the properties of conductivity (transmission of nerve impulses) and irritability (reaction to nerve impulses). Each neuron comprises a cell body (*soma*), an *axon* (a long projection that conducts impulses away from the cell body), and usually one or more *dendrites* (branching projections that conduct impulses toward the cell body).

a. Components of the cell body of a neuron. The cell body of a neuron is surrounded by a *cell membrane*, which encloses the cytoplasm. Within the cell body is the *nucleus*, which contains large quantities of deoxyribonucleic acid (DNA). Located within the nucleus is the *nucleolus*, which contains ribonucleic acid (RNA). Also within the cell body are *mitochondria*, which provide energy for the cell. The *Golgi apparatus* stores secretory substances, synthesizes carbohydrates, and forms digestive substances. The *endoplasmic reticulum* serves as a transport/communication system within the cell. Finally, *Nissl bodies*, which are composed of endoplasmic reticulum and ribosomes, synthesize proteins. Figure 1-1 illustrates a neuron and some of its structures.

Figure 1-1 *Typical motor neuron and some of its structures*

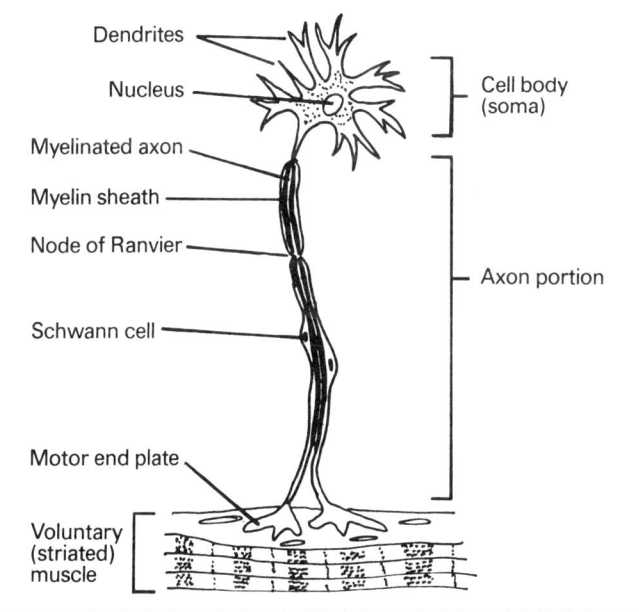

b. Structure of axons and dendrites. Structurally, dendrites contain Nissl bodies, branch profusely, and extend short distances. Axons, on the other hand, extend long distances, branch at their termination, and lack Nissl bodies. A *myelin sheath* surrounds many axons, usually larger neuron fibers. Composed of a lipid substance and formed by *Schwann cells*, the myelin sheath acts as an insulator for the conduction of impulses. Surrounding the myelin sheath is an outer layer called the *neurolemma*, which is necessary for axon regeneration. The segmented myelin sheath is interrupted by spaces called *nodes of Ranvier* (Figure 1-1).

c. Classification of neurons. Neurons can be unipolar, containing only an axon; bipolar, containing one axon and one dendrite; or, most commonly, multipolar, containing one axon and many dendrites (Figure 1-1).

C. Conduction of nerve impulses

1. Resting membrane potential

The state when the neuron is at rest and not conducting an impulse is called *resting membrane potential*. There is a positive electrical charge outside the cell membrane as a result of a greater concentration of sodium ions (Na^+) and chloride ions (Cl^-) in the interstitial space. Inside the cell is a negative electrical charge, with high concentrations of potassium ions (K^+) and organic protein materials.

2. Action potential of the neuron

Application of a sufficient stimulus causes conduction of an impulse, which in turn changes the cell membrane's permeability to certain ions. Sodium enters the cell and potassium goes into the interstitial space. This exchange of positive and negative charges is called *depolarization*. The action potential is conducted along the neuron and, in turn, from one neuron to the next. The change back to the resting, or polarized, state is called *repolarization*.

3. Saltatory conduction

In myelinated fibers, the action potential jumps from one node of Ranvier to the next. Saltatory conduction increases the velocity of the impulse and conserves energy.

4. Synapse

The synapse is the junction between a presynaptic terminal of an axon of one neuron and the soma or dendrite of another. As the action potential reaches the presynaptic terminal, the terminal's synaptic vesicles release either excitatory or inhibitory neurotransmitters (see Section 5) into the *synaptic cleft*, a microscopic space between the presynaptic terminal and the receptor area of the postsynaptic membrane of the adjacent neuron. The postsynaptic membrane contains specialized receptors for the transmitter substance.

5. Neurotransmitters

The two types of neurotransmitters are termed *excitatory* and *inhibitory*. A given neuron can secrete only one type. Among the several excitatory transmitters, acetylcholine is the most common. Others are norepinephrine, dopamine, and serotonin. Inhibitory transmitters include glycine and gamma-aminobutyric acid.

6. Excitation and inhibition of the postsynaptic membrane

The release of an excitatory transmitter causes local depolarization of the postsynaptic membrane and resulting transmission of the impulse. An inhibitory transmitter, on the other hand, causes the postsynaptic membrane to become less permeable to sodium ions. Its resultant hyperpolarized state renders it more stable and less excitable.

7. Inactivation of the neurotransmitter

Enzymes can break down or inactivate neurotransmitters, either at the receptor site of the postsynaptic membrane or in the synaptic cleft. Such enzymes include cholinesterase, monoamine oxidase (MAO), and catechol O-methyltransferase (COMT). Another mode of inactivation is the *reuptake mechanism*, which allows the neurotransmitter to be taken back up into the presynaptic terminal.

D. Divisions of the nervous system

The nervous system comprises the *central nervous system*, containing the brain and spinal cord, and the *peripheral nervous system*, containing the cranial nerves, the spinal nerves, and the *autonomic nervous system*.

E. Central nervous system
1. Bony structures

Eight bones make up the skull, or cranium, which encloses the brain (Figure 1-2): the frontal bone, occipital bone, sphenoid bone, ethmoid bone, two temporal bones, and two parietal bones. The bones of the skull join to form lines called *sutures*.

The 33 vertebrae of the spine protect the spinal cord. There are seven cervical vertebrae, 12 thoracic vertebrae, five lumbar vertebrae, five sacral vertebrae fused into one, and five coccygeal vertebrae fused into one. Fibrocartilaginous *intervertebral discs* separate the vertebrae.

Figure 1-2 *Side view of the skull*

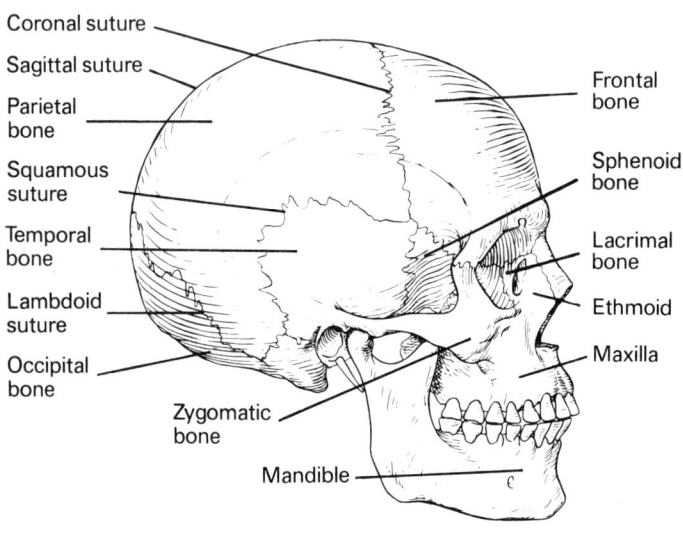

2. Meninges

Three membranes, the *meninges*, cover the brain and spinal cord:

a. Dura mater. The outermost layer of the meninges, the *dura mater*, is a tough, leathery, double-layered membrane. A fold of the dura, the *tentorium cerebelli*, separates the cerebellum and brain stem from the cerebral hemispheres.

b. Arachnoid. The middle membrane is called the *arachnoid* for its thin, spider web-like appearance.

c. Pia mater. The innermost meningeal layer, the *pia mater*, is a thin, vascular membrane that covers the entire surface of the brain and spinal cord.

3. Meningeal spaces

a. Epidural space. The *epidural space* describes the area between the skull and the outermost dural layer.

b. Subdural space. The *subdural space* is located between the inner dural and arachnoid membranes.

c. Subarachnoid space. Found between the arachnoid and pia, the *subarachnoid space* contains cerebrospinal fluid.

4. Cerebrum

The cerebral cortex is composed of pairs of lobes. The *great longitudinal fissure* divides it into right and left cerebral hemispheres.

a. Frontal lobe. The *frontal lobe* contains the *primary motor area* (Figure 1-3), including the premotor cortex, or motor association area, Broca's area, which is responsible for motor speech, and a large association area related to behavior and judgment.

b. Parietal lobe. Posterior to the central sulcus lies the *parietal lobe*. Within the lobe, the *primary sensory cortex* analyzes gross aspects of sensation. *Sensory association areas* analyze specific characteristics of sensory input. The parietal lobe also provides spatial orientation, an awareness of body parts, and analysis of spatial relationships.

Figure 1-3 *Side view of the brain, showing principal functional areas*

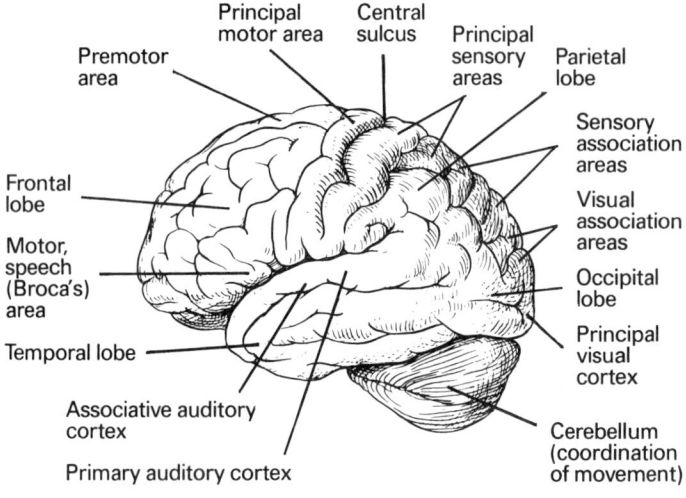

c. Temporal lobe. Integration of somatic, auditory, and visual association areas takes place within the *temporal lobe*.

d. Occipital lobe. The *occipital lobe* contains the *primary visual receptive area*, which permits vision. Also inside the lobe are the *visual association areas*, which allow understanding of the significance of what is seen.

5. Diencephalon

Figure 1-4 shows some of the internal structures of the brain and brain stem.

a. Thalamus. The *thalamus* processes impulses and relays them to the cerebral cortex. It is also responsible for pain awareness.

b. Epithalamus. The epithalamus is concerned with growth and development. It also regulates the primitive reflex that calls for the acquisition of food.

Figure 1-4 *Medial section of the brain and brain stem*

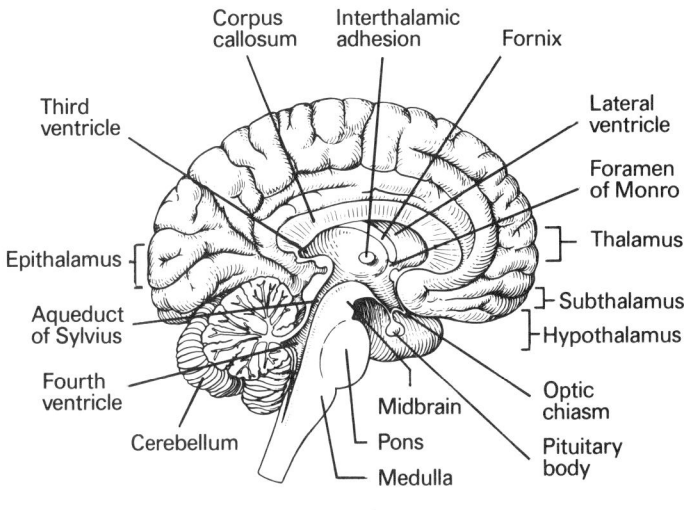

c. Hypothalamus. The *hypothalamus* has many functions: temperature control, water metabolism, appetite control, regulation of visceral and somatic activities, and physical expression of emotions. The hypothalamus also regulates pituitary secretions and is responsible for part of the sleep-wakefulness cycle.

d. Subthalamus. The function of the *subthalamus* is related to that of the basal ganglia.

6. Basal ganglia

The *basal ganglia* are concerned with motor control of fine body movements.

7. Pituitary gland

At the base of the brain, within a bony cavity called the *sella turcica*, lies the *pituitary gland*. The anterior pituitary, or *adenohypophysis*, secretes six hormones: growth hormone, adrenal-stimulating hormone, thyroid-stimulating hormone, prolactin, follicle-stimulating hormone, and luteinizing hormone. The posterior pituitary, or *neurohypophysis*, secretes antidiuretic hormone and oxytocin.

8. Cerebellum

The *cerebellum* is located in the posterior fossa (Figures 1-3 and 1-4). The cerebellum coordinates balance, movement, and the actions of muscle groups. It also controls fine movement.

9. Brain stem

The brain stem is comprised of the *midbrain, pons,* and *medulla* (Figure 1-4).

a. Midbrain. The midbrain, which lies between the diencephalon and the pons, contains the nuclei of cranial nerves III and IV. It also contains motor and sensory pathways and interconnections with the brain stem, cortex, and spinal cord.

b. Pons. Located between the midbrain and medulla is the *pons*, which contains the nuclei of cranial nerves V through VIII. The pons forms a bridge for nerve pathways between the midbrain, cerebellum, and medulla.

c. Medulla. The medulla, a continuation of the spinal cord, connects with the pons and the cerebellum. The medulla contains ascending and descending pathways as well as the nuclei of cranial nerves IX through XII. Also within the medulla is part of the reticular formation (see below).

10. Specialized systems of the brain

The collection of diffuse neurons in the brain stem and diencephalon is called the *reticular formation*. It provides continuous impulses that maintain the muscle tone that supports the body. Beginning in the lower brain and traveling up to the cerebral cortex is the *reticular activating system*. It controls sleep, wakefulness, and the ability to direct attention toward specific areas of the conscious mind.

11. Ventricular system

The ventricles are spaces within the brain that contain cerebrospinal fluid (Figure 1-4). Two lateral ventricles lie within the cerebral hemispheres. A third ventricle, below the lateral ventricles, is separated from them by the *foramen of Monro*. The fourth ventricle, which lies below the third, is separated from it by the *aqueduct of Sylvius*.

12. Cerebrospinal fluid

Cerebrospinal fluid (CSF) is a clear, colorless, odorless solution that fills the ventricles and subarachnoid space. Composed of water, protein, oxygen, carbon dioxide, electrolytes, and glucose, CSF acts as a shock absorber. When a person is recumbent, CSF normally tests at 60 to 180 mm of water pressure. The adult body contains approximately 125 to 150 ml of CSF.

13. Production, absorption, and flow of cerebrospinal fluid

Cerebrospinal fluid is formed by the *choroid plexus* — small capillary vessels in the ventricles. Up to 840 ml are secreted daily. Circulation of CSF is completed when it's reabsorbed by the *arachnoid villi* — projections from the subarachnoid space into the venous sinuses of the brain.

CSF flows from the lateral ventricles into the third ventricle via the foramen of Monro, then through the aqueduct of Sylvius to the fourth ventricle. It moves into the central canal and subarachnoid space to circulate around the spinal cord and brain.

14. Cerebral circulation

Blood to the brain is supplied by two pairs of arteries — the vertebral arteries and the internal carotid arteries — at a rate of approximately 750 ml/minute. The vertebral arteries supply blood to the posterior portion of the brain, including the brain stem. The *internal carotid arteries*, supply blood to most of the hemispheres except the occipitals, the basal ganglia, and the upper two-thirds of the diencephalon. The *circle of Willis* (Figure 1-5) is a ring of vessels formed by the branches of the vertebral and internal carotid arteries found

Figure 1-5 *Circle of Willis*

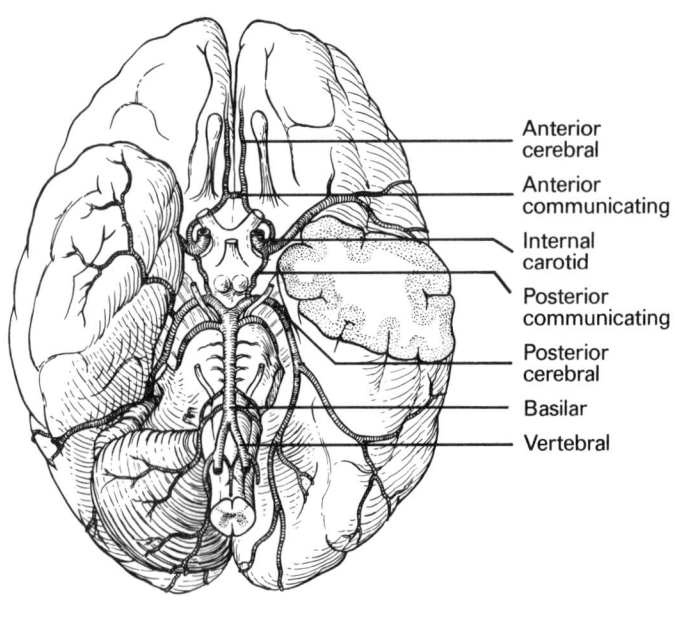

- Anterior cerebral
- Anterior communicating
- Internal carotid
- Posterior communicating
- Posterior cerebral
- Basilar
- Vertebral

at the base of the skull and is divided into anterior and posterior circulation.

15. Venous drainage

Veins of the brain are unique in that they have no valves and drain into large venous channels called *dural sinuses*, which lie between the two layers of dura. The *superior longitudinal sinus* receives blood from the veins of the convexity of the brain. Veins from the inferior surface of the brain drain *into* the *cavernous sinus*. The *inferior longitudinal sinus* receives venous drainage from the medial surface.

16. Blood-brain barrier

A mechanism called the blood-brain barrier, which occurs at the capillary level, inhibits certain chemicals from passing from the bloodstream into the brain and spinal cord.

17. Spinal cord

The cylindrical *spinal cord* connects the brain and peripheral nerves. It contains sensory and motor conducting pathways. The cord extends from the first cervical level to an area between the first and second vertebrae. It then tapers to form the *conus medullaris*. Meninges and nerve roots continue below the cord. The *filum terminale*, a thin filament of pia, continues to the second coccygeal segment.

a. Cross-section of the spinal cord. On cross-section, the cord looks like a butterfly- or H-shaped area of gray matter surrounded by white matter (Figure 1-6). The amount of gray matter varies, depending on the cord level. The H-shaped area is divided into anterior horns, posterior horns, and a connecting bar that contains the central canal. The gray matter contains cell bodies, unmyelinated or lightly myelinated nerve fibers, and glial cells.

The white matter, which contains myelinated and nonmyelinated nerve fibers, is divided into funiculi. Two *posterior funiculi* are divided by the posterior median septum. The white matter between the dorsal and ventral nerve roots is called the lateral funiculus. Two *anterior funiculi* are divided by the anterior median fissure and bordered by the ventral root fibers.

Figure 1-6 *Cross-section of spinal cord*

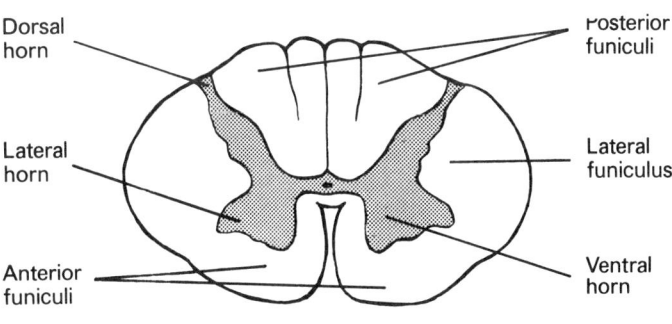

ANATOMY AND PHYSIOLOGY OF THE NERVOUS SYSTEM

b. Sensory (ascending) tracts. Sensory tracts are ascending pathways that relay impulses from the periphery to the brain. There are several major tracts of this type. The *posterior columns* are responsible for proprioception and deep sensory impulses. The fibers of this tract cross over (decussate) in the medulla. The *anterior spinothalamic tract* is located in the anterior funiculus. The fibers of this tract cross to the opposite side of the spinal cord at entrance level. Impulses relayed include direct touch, muscle sense, tickling, itching, and sexual feeling. The lateral spinothalamic tract, whose fibers decussate in the spinal cord, is found in the lateral funiculus. This tract transmits impulses of pain and temperature. The *posterior* and *anterior spinocerebellar* tracts, also found in the lateral funiculus, transmit impulses of muscle tone, unconscious muscle sense, and muscle coordination. The fibers of these tracts do not cross.

c. Motor (descending) tracts. The motor tracts originate in the cerebral cortex. There are several major descending tracts. The *corticospinal (pyramidal) tract* (Figure 1-7) transmits impulses of conscious muscle contraction. Ninety percent of the fibers of this tract decussate in the medulla to become the *lateral corticospinal tract*. The remaining fibers remain uncrossed and become the *anterior corticospinal tract*. The *corticorubrospinal tract* relays impulses of unconscious muscle coordination. Fibers cross before descending and are found in the lateral white matter. The *corticoreticulospinal tract* modifies and coordinates skeletal muscle activity. Fibers originate in the pons and travel down the anterior funiculi. The *vestibulospinal tract* assists in muscle tone maintenance and equilibrium. Fibers originate in the medulla and descend uncrossed.

F. The peripheral nervous system

1. Cranial nerves

The 12 pairs of cranial nerves are usually identified by Roman numerals. The function of each cranial nerve can be sensory, motor, or both, as well as autonomic.

Figure 1-7 *The pyramidal tract (reproduced, with permission, from Chaffee and Lytle: Basic Physiology and Anatomy, 4th ed. Philadelphia: Lippincott, 1980)*

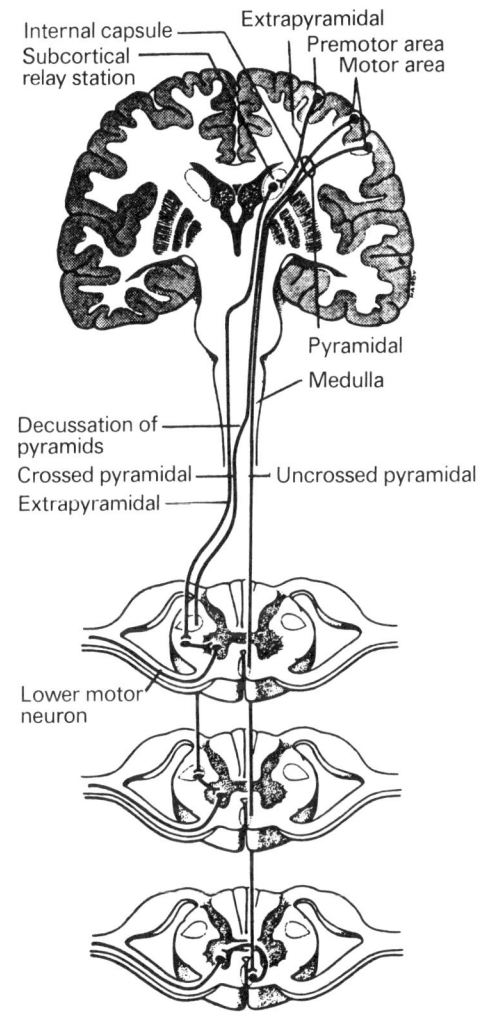

a. Olfactory nerve (I) (sensory). This nerve, which is responsible for the sense of smell, transmits from the nose to the frontal lobes.

b. Optic nerve (II) (sensory). The optic nerve is responsible for eyesight. It transmits from the retina of the eye to the occipital lobes.

c. Oculomotor nerve (III) (motor and autonomic). This nerve innervates four of the six muscles of eye movement, raises the eyelids, and constricts the pupils.

d. Trochlear nerve (IV) (motor). The trochlear nerve controls the muscle of the eyeball that rotates the eye downward and out.

e. Trigeminal nerve (V) (motor and sensory). This nerve carries the sensations of pain, temperature, and touch from the face, scalp, and nasal and oral cavities. It also controls the muscles of chewing and the corneal reflex.

f. Abducens nerve (VI) (motor). This nerve controls the muscle that rotates the eyeball outward.

g. Facial nerve (VII) (sensory and motor). The facial nerve innervates the muscles of facial expression. It's also responsible for the sense of taste on the anterior two-thirds of the tongue.

h. Acoustic nerve (VIII) (sensory). The acoustic nerve has two branches. The cochlear branch is responsible for hearing; the vestibular branch, for balance.

i. Glossopharyngeal nerve (IX) (sensory, motor, and autonomic). The glossopharyngeal nerve carries sensation from the pharynx and the sensation of taste from the posterior one-third of the tongue. It controls secretion of saliva and, with the vagus nerve, the act of swallowing. It is responsible for the gag reflex.

j. Vagus nerve (X) (sensory, motor, and autonomic). The vagus nerve innervates organs of the thoracic and abdominal cavities. It is responsible for sensation in the throat and larynx, the act of swallowing, and voice production.

k. Spinal accessory nerve (XI) (motor). The spinal accessory nerve is responsible for the ability to shrug the shoulders and to rotate the head.

l. Hypoglossal nerve (XII) (motor). The hypoglossal nerve regulates the tongue movement necessary for speech and swallowing.

2. Spinal nerves

The 31 pairs of spinal nerves include eight pairs of cervical nerves, 12 pairs of thoracic nerves, five pairs of lumbar nerves, five pairs of sacral nerves, and one pair of coccygeal nerves. The cervical and thoracic nerves emerge horizontally, whereas the lumbar, sacral, and coccygeal nerves descend from the point of origin (Figure 1-8). The sacral and coccygeal nerves form a group of nerves below the spinal cord called the *cauda equina*.

Figure 1-8 *The spinal nerves (reproduced, with permission, from Chaplin and Demers: Primer of Neurology and Neurophysiology. New York: Wiley, 1978)*

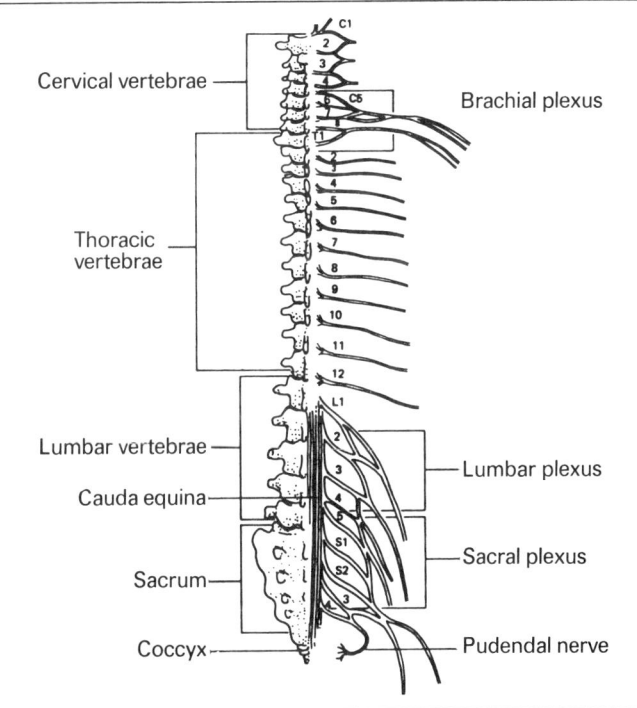

a. Dorsal roots. The dorsal roots of the spinal nerves convey sensory (afferent) impulses from various sensory receptors to the spinal cord. The skin segments innervated by the dorsal roots are called *dermatomes* (Figure 1-9). Impulses are transmitted via the dorsal roots to the dorsal ganglia, where the sensory cell bodies are located.

Figure 1-9 *Dermatomes, anterior and posterior views (reproduced, with permission, from Chaplin and Demers: Primer of Neurology and Neurophysiology. New York: Wiley, 1978)*

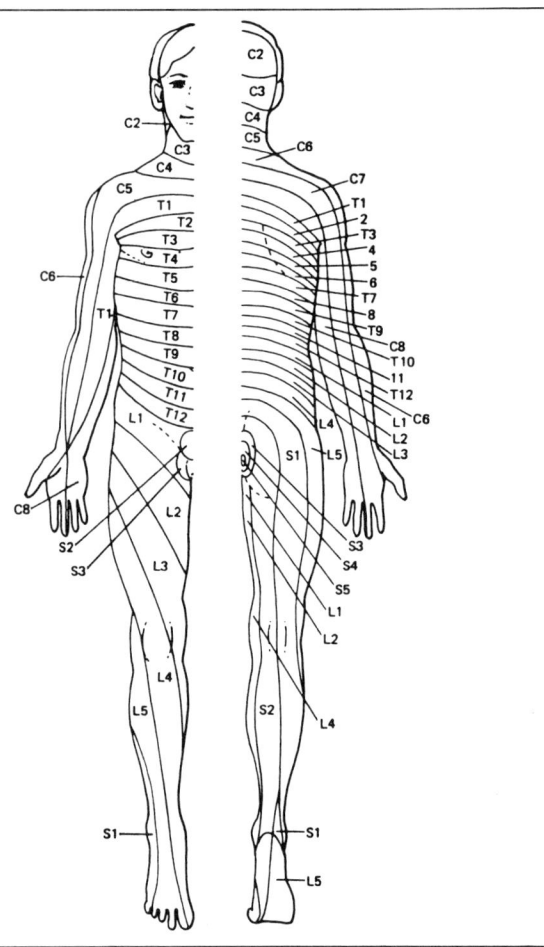

b. Ventral roots. The ventral roots of the spinal nerves transmit motor (efferent) impulses from the spinal cord to the muscles and glands of the body.

c. Plexuses. There are four major *plexuses*, or networks, of interwoven spinal nerves (Figure 1-8). The *cervical plexus* comprises the first four cervical nerves. It innervates the back of the head, the neck, and the shoulders, and gives rise to the phrenic nerve. The *brachial plexus*, which consists of the last four cervical nerves and the first thoracic nerve, innervates the upper extremities.

The *lumbar plexus* is made up of the first four lumbar nerves and may also include the 12th thoracic nerve. It innervates the lower trunk and part of the lower extremities and gives rise to the femoral nerve. Finally, the *sacral plexus* consists of the last two lumbar and first three sacral nerves. This plexus innervates the lower extremities and gives rise to the sciatic nerve.

d. Reflex arc. Simple reflexes, such as the knee jerk, represent simple nervous circuits in the spinal cord and do not involve the higher brain centers. A *three-neuron reflex arc* (Figure 1-10) involves a sensory receptor, a sensory neuron,

Figure 1-10 *Three-neuron reflex arc (reproduced, with permission, from Jacob, Francone, and Lossow: Structure and Function in Man, 5th ed. Philadelphia: Saunders, 1982)*

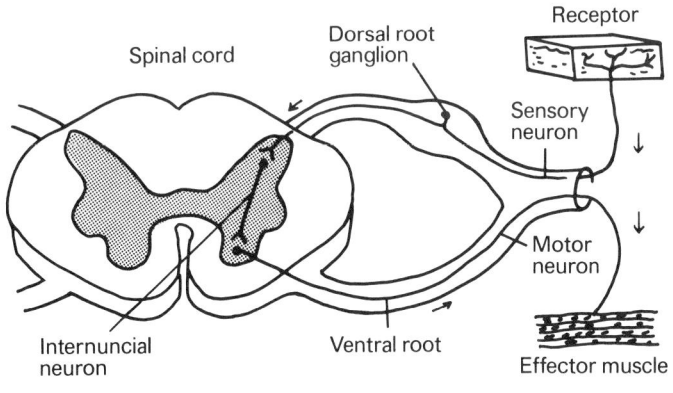

Figure 1-11 *The sympathetic nervous system (reproduced, with permission, from Miller, Drakontides, and Leavell: Kimber-Gray-Stackpole's Anatomy and Physiology, 17th ed. New York: Macmillan, 1977)*

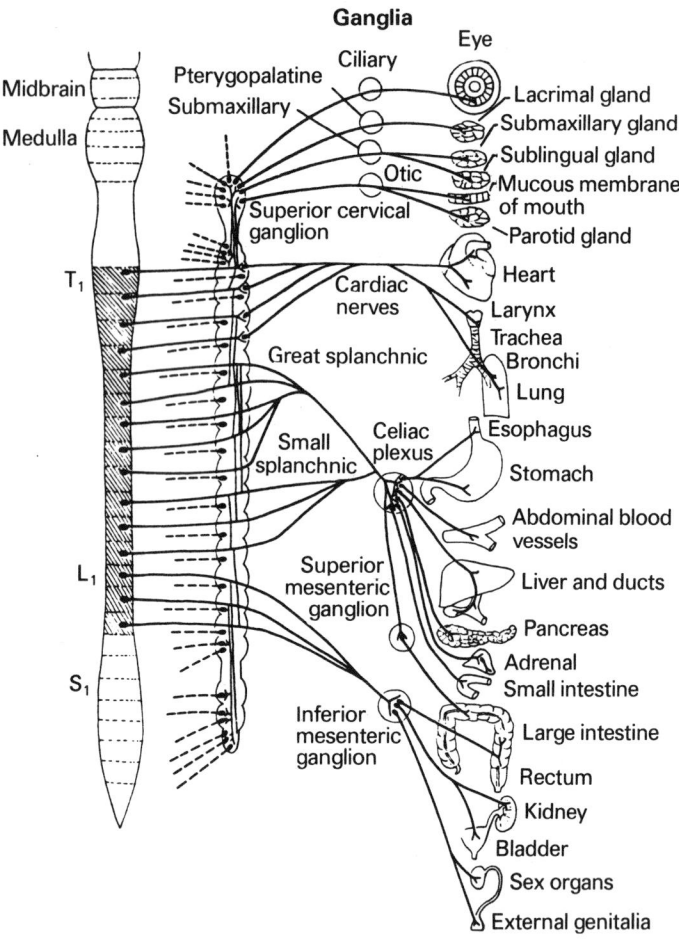

an association neuron (interneuron) within the spinal cord, and a motor neuron. The sensory receptor detects the stimuli that travel to the spinal cord by means of a sensory neuron. This activates interneurons, which in turn activate motor neurons to produce a motor response such as drawing away from a source of pain.

With *two-neuron reflex arcs*, the sensory neuron synapses directly with motor neurons in the spinal cord. The knee jerk is one example.

3. Autonomic nervous system

The autonomic nervous system regulates and coordinates vital visceral activities. It innervates three types of effector cells: involuntary (smooth) muscle cells, cardiac muscle cells, and glandular (secretory) cells. The system's two divisions are the sympathetic nervous system and the parasympathetic nervous system.

a. Sympathetic nervous system. The sympathetic nervous system comprises a chain of ganglia (groups of cell bodies) and nerves on either side of the spinal cord (Figure 1-11). The chain extends from the cervical through the lumbar region. Because preganglionic neurons originate in the thoracic and upper lumbar segments of the spinal cord, this system is referred to as the thoracolumbar division. The neurotransmitter of preganglionic neurons, which terminate in the sympathetic ganglia, is acetylcholine; therefore, the preganglionic fibers are *cholinergic*.

The postganglionic neurons originate at the sympathetic ganglia and terminate in involuntary muscle tissue or glandular tissue. The postganglionic neurons' neurotransmitter is norepinephrine; thus, the fibers are *adrenergic*. During stress, the adrenergic division acts as a total unit to produce a widespread response. The efferent response to sympathetic stimulation is summarized in Table 1-1.

b. Parasympathetic nervous system. The preganglionic fibers of this system leave the brain stem via cranial nerves III, VII, IX, and X, and exit from the spinal cord via the second, third, and fourth sacral segments (Figure 1-12). Therefore, this division is also called the craniosacral division. The

TABLE 1-1

EFFERENT RESPONSES OF THE AUTONOMIC NERVOUS SYSTEM

Structure and function	Sympathetic division	Parasympathetic division
Eye		
Iris	Dilates pupils	Constricts pupils
Ciliary muscle	Inhibits, flattens lenses	Stimulates bulging of lenses
Heart	Increases rate	Decreases rate
	Increases force of contraction	
Blood vessels		
Coronary arteries	Dilates	Constricts
Skeletal muscle	Dilates	No effect
Abdominal viscera and skin	Constricts	No effect
Blood pressure	Increases	Decreases
Bronchi	Dilates	Constricts
Respiratory rate	Increases	Decreases
Digestive system		
Salivary gland secretion	Thickens saliva	Increases watery saliva
Peristalsis	Decreases	Increases
Digestive secretions	Decreases	Increases
Liver		
Bile secretion	Decreases	Increases
Glycogen to glucose	Increases	No effect
Bladder		
Muscle walls	Relaxes	Contracts
Sphincters	Contracts	Relaxes
Adrenal glands	Increases secretion	No effect
Skin		
Sweat glands	Increases	No effect
Pilomotor muscles	Contracts	No effect

preganglionic fibers are long, and the postganglionic neurons lie close to the innervated organs. Both pre- and postganglionic neurons release acetylcholine, making the parasympathetic fibers cholinergic. Because acetylcholine is rapidly deactivated by cholinesterase, parasympathetic responses tend to be brief. Table 1-1 describes parasympathetic responses.

Figure 1-12 *The parasympathetic nervous system (reproduced, with permission, from Miller, Drakontides, and Leavell: Kimber-Gray-Stackpole's Anatomy and Physiology, 17th ed. New York: Macmillan, 1977)*

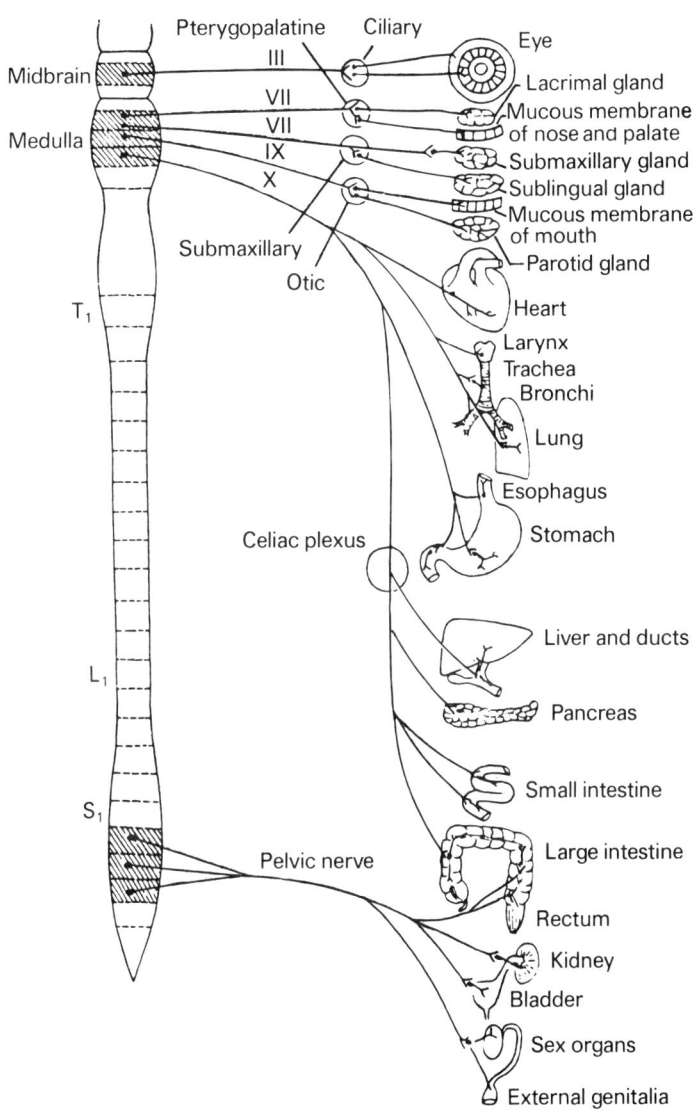

QUIZ

1. The part of the neuron that brings a stimulus into the cell is:
   a. An axon
   b. A neurilemma
   c. A dendrite
   d. A neurofibril

2. Neurotransmitters can be inactivated by which of the following mechanisms?
   a. Reuptake mechanism
   b. Receptor mechanism
   c. Biosynthesis mechanism
   d. Refractory mechanism

3. The three membranes surrounding the brain and spinal cord are the _____.

4. The _____ is the area of the brain concerned with balance, muscle tone, and coordination of fine movement.

5. CSF flows from the lateral ventricles through the _____ into the _____ ventricle, then through the _____ into the _____ ventricle.

6. CSF is reabsorbed by projections of the dura called _____.

7. Sensory and motor pathways run through the _____ matter of the spinal cord.

8. Match each cranial nerve with its function:

Olfactory _____	**a.** Laryngeal function
Optic _____	**b.** Muscles of the eye
Oculomotor _____	**c.** Tongue muscles
Trochlear, abducens _____	**d.** Facial expression
Trigeminal _____	**e.** Swallowing
Facial _____	**f.** Smell
Acoustic _____	**g.** Hearing
Glossopharyngeal _____	**h.** Rotation of head
Vagus _____	**i.** Eyesight
Spinal accessory _____	**j.** Sensation of face
Hypoglossal _____	**k.** Pupil size

9. The neurotransmitter released by the parasympathetic preganglionic and postganglionic neurons is _____. This neurotransmitter is deactivated by _____.

10. The neurotransmitter of the sympathetic postganglionic neuron is _____.

ANSWERS

1. c.

2. a.

3. Meninges.

4. Cerebellum.

5. Foramen(ina) of Monro; third; aqueduct of Sylvius; fourth.

6. Arachnoid villi.

7. White.

8. Olfactory—**f.** Optic—**i.** Oculomotor—**k.** Trochlear, abducens—**b.** Trigeminal—**j.** Facial—**d.** Acoustic—**g.** Glossopharyngeal—**e.** Vagus—**a.** Spinal accessory—**h.** Hypoglossal—**c.**

9. Acetylcholine; cholinesterase.

10. Norepinephrine.

CHAPTER

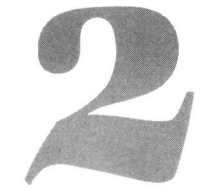

The Neurologic History

OBJECTIVES

After completing this chapter, you will be able to:
1. *Make pertinent neurologic observations during the patient interview*
2. *Analyze each presenting neurologic symptom according to eight specific elements*
3. *Evaluate selected neurologic symptoms according to their specific criteria*
4. *Obtain a significant history through a review of systems*
5. *Obtain a pertinent personal and family history.*

A. Introduction

Patient evaluation requires an accurate and complete neurologic history. It not only provides facts on the nature of the neurologic dysfunction but also helps determine the effect of the dysfunction on a patient's ability to handle everyday activities. From this information, you can formulate a nursing diagnosis and care plan.

But taking a history isn't easy. It needs skill, time, understanding, and patience. For example, you must allow the patient to relate the account of his illness in *his own words* and, if necessary, help him to describe his symptoms in the most precise terms. Obviously, you must gauge the precise meaning of the details given and, further, direct the interview by asking pertinent questions at the right moments.

Good history-taking technique calls for study and repeated trials. These guidelines will help you, but you'll want to adapt them to the setting, the patient's needs, and the time you have available.

B. Observations during the neurologic history

As you take the patient's history, use the opportunity to observe both his motor abilities and mental status. The information you gain from careful observation will be useful when you perform the neurologic assessment.

1. Observation of motor status

When the patient walks into the room, observe his gait. Are abnormal characteristics present? Observe his posture as he walks and sits. Is it straight or bent over? Does he lean to one side? Do his actions appear coordinated? Do you see any involuntary movements, such as tics, tremors, or fasciculations? Does the patient appear restless? Is there any indication of paralysis? If you observe abnormalities in motor abilities during the interview, make a mental note to examine those areas carefully when performing your physical assessment.

2. Observation of mental status

While talking with the patient, note his emotional state. Does he appear alert, apathetic, animated, or irritable? Is his attitude euphoric, depressed, flippant, hostile, or suspicious? Does he pay attention, or does his mind appear to wander? Does he forget your questions? Are his answers appropriate and logical? Does he respond within a reasonable period of time, or too slowly?

Note whether the patient's discussion indicates orientation to person, time, and place. Does his memory seem intact? Does he remember recent events as well as those that have happened in the past? Again, make note of any abnormalities that will require further investigation.

C. The interview
1. Statistical data

It's essential to know the patient's name, sex, age, date and place of birth, residence, marital status, and occupation. Usually this information is found on the patient's chart, making repeated questioning in this area unnecessary. It's also important to determine whether the patient is right- or left-handed.

2. Presenting complaint

This is a detailed account of the patient's problem given in his own words. Ask the patient why he is seeking medical help. If he is unable to communicate, obtain the necessary information from a family member or other reliable source.

3. History of the present illness

Obtain a chronological account of each symptom the patient exhibits. Then, in order to analyze the symptoms further, question the patient according to these eight criteria:

1. Character of the symptom — how the symptom feels, and its intensity.

2. Date of first occurrence.

3. Mode of onset. — abrupt, or gradual

4. Usual time of onset, if symptom isn't constant

5. Precipitating factors — for instance, an action, substance, or emotion

6. Factors that alleviate or increase the complaint

7. Duration of the symptom — constant or intermittent

8. Progression or regression of the symptom

4. Analysis of complaints

Specific and detailed questioning regarding each symptom is necessary for a complete picture of the problem. Here are some common neurologic symptoms, with guidelines for obtaining necessary information on each:

a. Pain. Ask the patient the exact location of his pain. Does it tend to radiate and, if so, where? Is the pain throbbing, boring, sharp, dull, lancinating, deep, or superficial? Constant or intermittent? Does anything tend to relieve the pain — for example, drugs, heat, or posture? What aggravates it: movement, climate, straining?

b. Headache. Ask the patient to describe the location of his headache. Is it generalized, or in one specific place (focal)? Is it on one side of the head (unilateral) or both sides (bilateral)? Does it feel like a band around his head?

Next, ask the patient to describe the character of the headache: dull, always steady, throbbing, boring, burning, griping, sharp, constricting, continuous, or paroxysmal. You may have to help the patient find the best words to describe his headache. Determine whether the headache is incapacitating: Does the patient have to lie down or can he go about his regular activities without difficulty?

Does the headache come on gradually or abruptly? How long does it usually last? How often does it occur during a day, a week, or a month? Does anything cause it to begin — for example, a certain food, movement, position, exercise, mental effort, stress, or mood? What helps it go away? Does anything else occur with the headache, such as nausea, vomiting, double vision, blurred vision, hemianopsia, syncope, vertigo, aphasia, drowsiness, or convulsions?

c. Convulsions/seizures. If the patient is suffering from a seizure disorder, an exact description of the attacks is necessary. You may need to obtain this information from a witness since the patient himself may be unaware of what occurs during seizures.

Ask the patient if there's anything that tends to bring on the seizure. Does he have an aura or other premonition of the attack? If so, what is it, and how long does it last? Ask the patient—or, if available, a witness—to describe his movement patterns during the attack. Is he flaccid or rigid, and is the movement in one part of the body (focal) or generalized? Are the movements tonic, clonic, or both? Are they bizarre and purposeless, or coordinated and purposeful? Is there loss of consciousness with the seizure and, if so, is it sudden or gradual?

During the attack is there any cyanosis, pallor, or flushing? Is there incontinence of urine or feces, frothing at the mouth, tongue biting, or other bodily injury?

After the seizure, does the patient regain consciousness immediately? Does he feel fatigue, sleepiness, confusion, muscular soreness, nausea, vomiting, or headache? Is there any weakness of a body part and, if so, what is its duration? Does the patient experience any numbness and/or tingling, disturbed speech, amnesia, or behavior changes?

Ask the patient whether the attacks occur most often during the day or during sleep. Are they related to sleep? Are they related to activity, stress, meals, presence of people, or menses? Have the attacks been present since birth, or did they develop during infancy, puberty, or adult life? Was there a history of illness or injury prior to the first attack?

d. Vertigo. Try to determine the exact nature of the patient's complaint of dizziness. Does the patient feel that *he* is moving or rotating (subjective vertigo), or does he experience *objects* moving in the environment (objective vertigo)? Direct your questioning to determine the nature, mode of onset, duration, frequency, severity, and direction of the vertigo. Is it related to posture or position change? Are any symptoms associated with it, such as ataxia, nausea, vomiting, tinnitus, deafness, or perspiration?

e. Disturbances of movement. If the patient relates a history of paralysis, paresis, atrophy, tremors, or ataxia, you should determine the time and mode of onset, location, severity, type, and progression of the problem. Also determine whether there is weakness, fatigue, stiffness, clumsiness, stumbling, staggering, or disturbances of equilibrium.

f. Disturbance of sensation. The patient who relates a history of numbness, paresthesias, itching, tingling, or burning requires careful questioning. Determine the location and distribution of the sensory problem. Does it radiate from the initial point of sensation? What was the mode of onset? What is the character, severity, incidence, duration, and frequency? Is it affected by rest, position, motion, or sleep? Are there other aggravating factors? Is the sensation accompanied by localized tenderness, muscle rigidity, or spasm? Are there other associated symptoms? How is the symptom alleviated or worsened?

g. Visual disturbances. Exact determination of the extent and type of any visual problem is important. Is the patient's problem dimness or blurring of vision? Does he have indistinct vision (scotomas)? Double vision (diplopia) or transient blindness? Is the patient experiencing visual field defects? Visual hallucinations? If so, ask him to describe them. Once you determine the exact type of visual problem, ask him about the date of occurrence, mode of onset, precipitating factors, duration, and progression or regression of the problem.

h. Auditory disturbances. Question the patient as to the exact nature of his auditory difficulty: tinnitus, deafness, or auditory hallucinations (if so, have him describe them). Does he experience any associated symptoms such as vertigo, unsteadiness, or disturbances of equilibrium? Again, question the patient according to the eight criteria previously mentioned.

i. Disturbances of other cranial nerve functions. Is the patient having any problems with his sense of smell or taste?

Is he experiencing numbness or paralysis of the face? Does he have difficulty speaking (dysarthria)? Has he experienced difficulty swallowing liquids or solids (dysphagia)?

j. Sleep disturbances or alterations of consciousness. Discuss with the patient whether he is experiencing excessive drowsiness, an increased need for sleep, or attacks of uncontrollable need for sleep. Does he have insomnia or other changes in his sleeping patterns? Does he experience periods of confusion, delirium, or stupor? Has the patient ever been in a coma?

k. Disturbances of speech or expression. Question the patient regarding any problem he may be having with speech. Does he have difficulty expressing himself? Has he noticed problems in writing or drawing? Does he have difficulty understanding what is said to him? Does he have problems comprehending what he reads? Determine the extent of any problem, if present.

l. Visceral symptoms. Problems with the autonomic nervous system manifest themselves with a variety of symptoms. Ask the patient whether he has noticed changes in thirst, appetite, or elimination. Has he been vomiting? If so, has the vomiting been projectile? Is it accompanied by nausea? Does he have diarrhea or constipation? Does he have any urinary problems such as retention, frequency, urgency, pain on urination, or incontinence? Has he noticed problems in potency or changes in libido? Is he experiencing excessive sweating or flushing?

m. Mental symptoms. Ask the patient whether he or his family have noticed any personality changes. Does he appear anxious or tense? Has he experienced memory problems? Does he have a history of delirium, confusion, alcohol or drug abuse, or "nervous breakdown"?

n. Head trauma. If the patient has suffered trauma to the head either just previously or in the past, question him or his family regarding the details of the accident. Was there loss of consciousness and, if so, what was the duration? Was there bleeding or clear fluid drainage (CSF) from the nose or ears? After the accident, was the patient confused or disoriented? Did he experience convulsions, amnesia, memory disturbances, or personality changes?

5. Significant past history

In addition to the neurologic history, an evaluation of the patient's medical history can help you better understand his symptoms, and enable you to put his overall health in perspective. Question the patient regarding his general health prior to his present illness. Is there a history of past illnesses, operations, accidents, or injuries? If so, what were the dates, nature of each, duration, and aftereffects? Were there any significant problems before, during, or after the patient's birth? Did he experience any early developmental difficulties? What was his progress in school?

6. Review of systems

Further questions regarding the patient's body systems may reveal significant information that may have been overlooked in the neurologic and past histories.

a. Eyes. Does the patient need glasses or contact lenses? For what reason? Has he experienced visual difficulties, diplopia, blindness, blurring, visual field defects, or scotomas? Has he noticed any pain, discharge, inflammation, or swelling of his eyes?

b. Nose. Does the patient get frequent colds? Does he have a history of sinus disease, allergic rhinitis, epistaxis, discharge, obstruction, or loss of the sense of smell?

c. Ears. Does the patient have hearing loss, pain, tinnitus, discharge, or vertigo?

d. Mouth and throat. Does the patient have a history of sore throat, difficulty in swallowing or talking, or sore gums or mouth? What is the condition of his teeth?

e. Heart and lungs. Question the patient about dyspnea, night sweats, coughing, production of sputum, hemoptysis, wheezing, asthma, bronchitis, emphysema, pneumonia, tuberculosis, chest pains, palpitations, orthopnea, tachycardia, edema, heart murmurs, or hypertension.

f. Stomach and intestines. What are the patient's eating habits? Has he noticed a recent weight change? Does he have a history of nausea, vomiting, heartburn, jaundice, abdominal pain, change in bowel habits, flatulence, constipation, or incontinence of stool? Ask the patient to describe his stools. Does he often need a laxative?

g. Genitourinary and reproductive function. Does the patient have a history of frequency, urgency, burning on urination, nocturia, urinary incontinence, retention, hematuria, or pyuria? Ask women to describe their menstrual history and any difficulties with menstruation, as well as the age of menopause, if applicable.

h. Orthopedic history. Discuss with the patient any problems he may have had with growth. Does he have any swelling, pain, or redness in his joints? Does he experience any limitation of movement, or back and leg pains?

i. Skin. Discuss any history of rashes, pruritus, scaling, or sweat disturbances.

j. Allergic history. Has the patient experienced any acute or chronic allergic rhinitis, bronchitis, food or drug intolerance, or pollen and dust sensitivity? How are his allergic reactions manifested?

7. Occupational history

Investigate the patient's on-the-job contact with toxins, heavy metals, fumes, silica, or industrial hazards. Does his job cause physical or mental strain?

8. Educational history

Ask the patient how many years he attended school. Did he have any learning difficulties or social problems at school?

9. Personality inventory

Has the patient or his family noticed any major personality changes? How would they describe his personality? Does the description correspond with your own observations? Does the patient appear concerned with his outward appearance? What is his attitude toward his body, health, and present illness? What is his family's attitude?

10. Personal habits

Does the patient use alcohol, tobacco, drugs, coffee, or tea, and how much? What is his daily routine, including sleep and bowel habits? Does he exercise? How easily is he fatigued?

11. Family history

What were the ages and causes of death—if any—of the patient's parents or siblings? Discuss their physical and mental health during life. What is the family's cultural and economic background?

QUIZ

1. You are preparing to obtain a complete neurologic history from Mr. S. As he walks into the room and sits down, you are able to make several observations regarding his motor status. List *four* aspects of the patient's motor status that you observed:

2. During your discussion with Mr. S, you note that he appears alert but slightly depressed. He is able to pay attention and answers questions appropriately and logically. You also observe two other aspects of his mental status:

3. Mr. S is complaining of tinnitus with no vertigo or unsteadiness. He states that the ringing is loud and present all the time. It began abruptly 1 month ago. Utilizing the eight criteria for analyzing a symptom, what other information would you obtain from Mr. S?

4. Mr. S also complains of headaches. The pain is throbbing on the right side of his head. The headaches began 2 months ago and he has had approximately two each week. What other information would you obtain from Mr. S about his headaches?

5. Which of the following questions would you include in obtaining a past medical history from Mr. S?

___ **a.** "Tell me about your health before this present problem."
___ **b.** "Do you smoke?"
___ **c.** "What do you do for a living?"
___ **d.** "Do you have any allergies?"
___ **e.** "Did you ever have any learning difficulties in school?"
___ **f.** "Are your parents alive?"
___ **g.** "Have you ever had any operations?"
___ **h.** "Do you ever have chest pain?"
___ **i.** "How is your eyesight?"
___ **j.** "Do you have frequent colds?"

6. During your investigation of the patient's occupational history, you should determine whether his job causes _____ or _____ strain.

7. An accurate educational history should include information on the presence of any _____ difficulties.

8. While obtaining a personality inventory, discuss with the patient his attitude toward his _____, _____, and _____ illness.

9. Inquiries into the patient's personal habits should include his use of _____, _____, drugs, coffee, and tea.

10. While discussing the family history, it is important to determine the age and cause of death of _____ and _____.

THE NEUROLOGIC HISTORY

ANSWERS

1. Gait, posture, coordination, presence of involuntary movements, presence of paralysis, restlessness.
2. Orientation, memory.
3. Precipitating factors; events that alleviate or increase the complaints; progression or regression of the symptom.
4. Time of onset, intensity, precipitating factors, duration, factors that alleviate or increase the pain, associated symptoms.
5. **a, e, g.**
6. Physical; mental.
7. Learning.
8. Body; health; present.
9. Alcohol; tobacco.
10. Parents; siblings.

CHAPTER

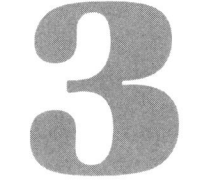

Assessment of the Neurologic Patient

OBJECTIVES

After completing this chapter, you will be able to:

1. Assess cognitive function

2. Assess sensory and motor integration

3. Assess the ability to communicate in spoken and written language

4. Evaluate cranial nerve function

5. Assess balance and coordination

6. Evaluate primary and discriminatory sensations

7. Identify motor abnormalities, including involuntary movements

8. Evaluate muscle size, tone, and strength

9. Assess deep tendon, superficial, and pathologic reflexes.

A. Rationale for neurologic assessment

Nursing assessment of the neurologic patient provides a data base – specifically, the means for planning nursing care and evaluating changes in your patient's condition. In addition, the time spent with a patient should establish rapport between you. He *does* want to get to know his nurse.

B. General observations

As you start the examination, observe the patient's appearance and behavior, and note anything that seems abnormal.

Note whether his clothing and grooming are appropriate. An unkempt appearance or inappropriate attire could indicate depression or a chronic brain disease. Evaluate the patient's mood by observing his facial expressions and physical movements, and by listening to him. Does he appear anxious, depressed, euphoric, angry, or hostile? Does he cry or laugh inappropriately? Is he able to cooperate with the exam?

While the patient is speaking, listen to the rate of his speech and the flow of his words. Can he speak clearly? Is his speech coherent and relevant? Note, too, whether the patient seems obsessed with a certain idea. Does he express inappropriate fears or paranoid feelings? Does he hallucinate?

C. Cognitive functions

You can make a rough determination of your patient's intellectual capability and memory by using the following questions and simple tests. Take the patient's educational and socioeconomic background into account.

1. Orientation to person, place, and time

Ask the patient his name, address, name of spouse or close family member, present location, time of day, day of the week, the month, the year, and season of the year. Phrase each question carefully to avoid any confusion.

2. Ability to follow commands

Ask the patient to perform a simple act, such as picking up a pencil. Increase the complexity by giving several commands at once. For example, ask him to pick up a pencil, raise his arms above his head, and close his eyes.

3. Calculations

First ask the patient to count backward from 100 in decrements of 7, and then ask him to perform some simple mathematical problems.

4. Abstract reasoning

Abstract reasoning can be tested by asking the patient the meaning of a proverb such as "A stitch in time saves nine."

5. Attention and concentration

Ask the patient to repeat a number series. Begin with two-digit numbers, then increase to numbers of three, four, five, etc. Then ask the patient to repeat a series backward. Normally, a person should be able to repeat correctly a series with five to eight digits forward and four to six backward.

6. Judgment

The ability to solve problems of daily life requires the ability to perceive the circumstances of various situations. Ask the patient what he would do if he lost his wallet, or if he found a sealed, stamped, addressed envelope on the street.

7. Memory

Immediate memory can be tested by giving the patient a list of three or four words and having him repeat them after you've finished. Then, about 5 minutes later, ask the patient to repeat the list. Remote memory can be determined by asking questions about past events such as "When were you married?"

D. Cerebral functions

Specific testing is required to assess the functioning of the cerebral cortex. Three areas are examined: sensory integration, motor integration, and language.

1. Sensory integration

The ability to recognize objects by sight, sound, and touch is a function of sensory integration. The inability to identify objects through the senses is called *agnosia*. There are four types of agnosia: visual, auditory, tactile, and spatial.

a. Visual agnosia. The inability to recognize common objects by sight is due to a lesion in the occipital lobe. To test for this cortical malfunction, ask the patient to point to objects in the room as you name them.

b. Auditory agnosia. The inability to recognize the meaning of common sounds is caused by a lesion in the temporal lobe. Test for this condition by asking the patient to close his eyes and identify various sounds he hears, such as a telephone bell or car horn.

c. Tactile agnosia (astereognosis). The inability to recognize common objects through the sense of touch is due to a lesion in the parietal lobe. To assess, ask the patient to close his eyes and identify an object (e.g., paper clip, key, pencil) that you've placed in his hand.

d. Spatial agnosia. Inability to identify body parts or understand their relationship to other parts is due to a lesion in the posterior inferior region of the parietal lobe. Can the patient identify different parts of his body? Does he know left from right?

2. Motor integration

In order for a person to carry out a skilled motor act, he must understand the goal, remember the directions, and have normal motor strength. The inability to carry out such an act in the absence of paralysis is called *apraxia*. To evaluate motor integration, ask the patient to do a simple task such as combing his hair or drinking from a cup.

3. Language

The inability to communicate orally or in writing is called *aphasia*. There are two types of aphasia: *Receptive aphasia* is the inability to understand the written or spoken word, while *expressive aphasia* is the inability to express one's thoughts by those means.

a. Ability to understand spoken words. First give the patient a simple command, such as "Close your eyes." If this is performed successfully, increase the complexity by asking him, "Go to the desk and pick up a book." Loss of this ability suggests a lesion in the temporal lobe.

b. Ability to understand written words. Ask the patient to follow a few simple commands that have been written on cards and shown to him. The inability to perform this test is due to a lesion in the parieto-occipital area.

c. Ability to express ideas orally. Ask the patient questions that require more than a "yes" or "no" answer. Inability to express ideas orally is due to a lesion in the inferior posterior frontal lobe.

d. Ability to express ideas in writing. Start by having the patient write his name and address, and then ask him to write a paragraph describing the day's events. An inability to do this is called *alexia*, and is due to a lesion in the posterior frontal area.

E. Cranial nerve functions

Continue your neurologic assessment by evaluating the 12 cranial nerves, as follows:

1. Olfactory nerve (I)

Before beginning this test, make sure the patient doesn't have a cold and his nasal passages are not blocked—conditions that would interfere with his sense of smell. Ask the patient to close one nostril. Place a vial containing a substance with a common scent such as coffee, cloves, or tobacco under the open nostril, and ask him to identify the odor. Repeat for the other nostril with a different substance. Loss of the sense of smell is called *anosmia*.

2. Optic nerve (II)

Evaluate each eye separately. You should first assess visual acuity and visual fields, and then conclude with an ophthalmoscopic examination.

a. Visual acuity. If a Snellen chart is available, have the patient sit 20 feet from the chart with one eye covered. Ask him to read the smallest line of print possible; test the other eye in the same way.

If no chart is available, ask the patient to read a few lines of small print of a newspaper at a set distance from the eye. If he is unable to see either that or larger print, hold up several fingers and ask him how many he sees.

b. Visual fields by confrontation. Sit directly in front of the patient, about 2 or 3 feet away, and ask him to cover one eye as you cover your opposite eye. Tell the patient to look at your nose while you look at his. Using your finger or a pen, bring it from the periphery into his field of vision, and ask him to tell you when he sees it. Compare the result with your own field of vision. Do this for all four quadrants of both eyes.

For more accuracy, a perimetry test performed by an ophthalmologist may be necessary. Tests for visual fields can reveal functional disturbances along the optic tract, from the retina to the occipital lobes.

c. Ophthalmoscopic examination. Your assessment of the optic nerve concludes with the ophthalmoscopic exam, which evaluates the optic discs, vessels, and periphery of the retina.

Darken the room and sit directly opposite the patient. Turn the upper dial of the ophthalmoscope to zero. With the patient looking straight ahead, hold the ophthalmoscope to your right eye with your right hand, about 12 inches away from the patient's right eye. Steady his head with your left hand.

Look through the viewer with your right eye and direct the beam of light to the patient's right pupil. You should see a red reflex. Now move in 3 inches away from the patient's eye. Adjust the focus of the ophthalmoscope to find the optic disc, which is located in the nasal area of the fundus. The optic disc is normally round or oval and lighter in color than the surrounding retina, with clearly defined margins. The depression in the center is the optic cup, which is normally whitish or pale yellow. Swollen margins and a reddish hue indicate that the optic disc is congested as a result of increased intracranial pressure. This condition is called *papilledema*.

Four main pairs of arteries and veins enter and leave the optic disc. The veins are slightly wider and darker than the arteries, and they pulsate. The arteries are brighter and reflect light.

The retina is normally reddish orange and somewhat lighter toward the nasal area. Examine it for hemorrhage or exudate.

Examine the macula last, as it's sensitive to light. The macula is located on the temporal side of the disc and is darker red. The center, the *fovea centralis*, will normally reflect light.

Using your left hand, repeat the procedure on the patient's left eye.

3. Oculomotor (III), trochlear (IV), and abducens (VI) nerves

These three cranial nerves are tested simultaneously, since they all interact to move the eyeball. The oculomotor nerve controls the muscles that allow the eye to look up, down, or medially, pupillary constriction and dilation, and the muscles of the upper eyelid. The trochlear nerve controls the muscles that move the eye downward and inward; the abducens nerve controls outward movement of the eyeball.

a. Ocular movements. To test extraocular movement, hold one finger about 18 inches from the patient's face, and ask him to follow it with his eyes, without moving his head. Observe the patient's eyes as you have him look straight ahead, then up and down; to the right, then up and down; and to the left, then up and down.

b. Pupils. Examine the pupils for size, shape, and equality. Then, in a darkened room, evaluate for pupillary constriction by shining a penlight into each eye. The opposite pupil should also constrict (consensual light reflex). Pupillary accommodation can be tested by asking the patient to focus on a pencil held about 18 inches from his nose and brought gradually closer to his eyes. The eyes should converge and the pupils constrict.

c. Eyelids. Observe for the presence of ptosis (drooping of the eyelids).

4. Trigeminal nerve (V)

This nerve transmits sensations of pain, temperature, and touch for the face, and controls the opening and closing of the jaw.

Test the patient's sensory function by asking him to close his eyes, and then lightly touch different parts of his face with a cotton ball, a pin, and test tubes of hot and cold

Figure 3-1 *Assessing trigeminal nerve (cranial nerve V) response to pain*

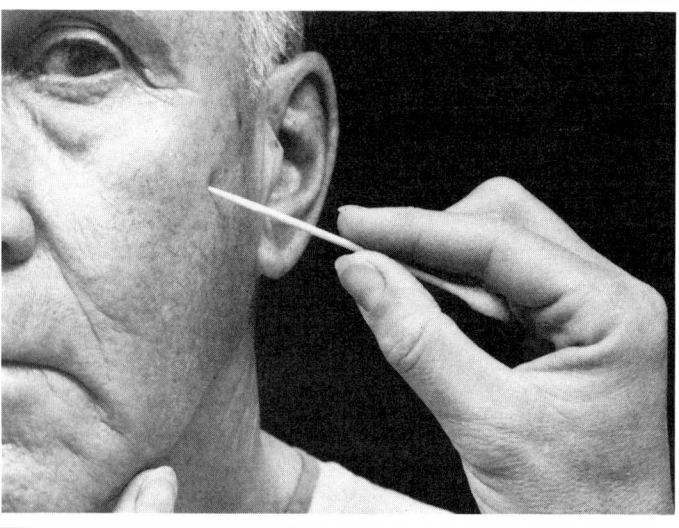

water (Figure 3-1). Ask him to tell you when and where he feels the sensation.

Test motor function by palpating the patient's temporal and masseter muscles with his jaws tightly closed. Note strength and muscle tone.

Finally, test the corneal reflex by noting whether the patient blinks when a wisp of cotton is lightly moved across the cornea (Figure 3-2).

5. Facial nerve (VII)

The facial nerve innervates the facial muscles and the taste receptors of the first two-thirds of the tongue. To examine, note any asymmetry or tics of the patient's face at rest and as he smiles, frowns, raises his eyebrows, whistles, and puffs out his cheeks. To test the strength of the eyelids, ask the patient to close his eyes and keep them closed as you try to open them.

Evaluate the sensory function of the facial nerve by placing some sugar on one side of the anterior portion of the

Figure 3-2 *Assessing trigeminal nerve (cranial nerve V) response to light touch (corneal reflex)*

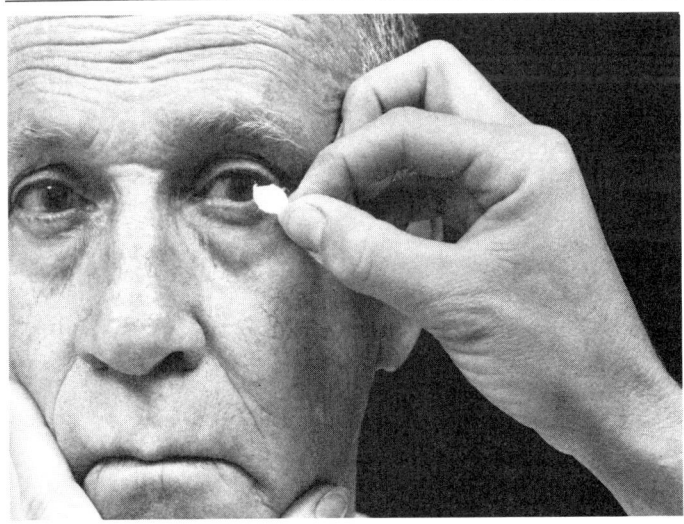

patient's tongue and asking him to identify the taste. After a sip of water, repeat the test on the other side, using salt. Discourage the patient from retracting his tongue or swallowing until he can identify the taste.

6. Acoustic nerve (VIII)

This nerve has two major divisions, cochlear (hearing) and vestibular (balance). The vestibular division usually is not tested unless the patient has a history of vertigo, tinnitus, or disturbed balance, in which case a physician would perform specialized tests.

To test hearing, hold a ticking watch at various distances from the ear to determine at what point the patient can no longer hear it. Repeat with the other ear.

To determine whether a hearing deficit is sensorineural or conductive, use the Weber test of lateral hearing. Place a vibrating tuning fork at the top of the skull or in the middle of the forehead and ask the patient whether the sound remains in the center or is referred to one side. If sound is heard more loudly in one ear, a conductive hearing loss may be present.

The Rinne test compares sound through air and bone conduction. Place a vibrating tuning fork on the mastoid process behind the ear and ask the patient to tell you when he can no longer hear it. Then hold the tuning fork near the ear canal until the sound is no longer audible. Sound conducted through air is normally heard longer than sound conducted through bone.

7. Glossopharyngeal (IX) and vagus (X) nerves

The glossopharyngeal nerve controls sensation in the pharynx and posterior third of the tongue, and motor functions of the pharynx. The vagus nerve controls swallowing and speaking, and regulates various autonomic functions of the lungs, heart, and digestive tract. (The autonomic functions are usually evaluated during a general physical examination.)

The glossopharyngeal nerve is checked by asking the patient to open his mouth and say "Ah." The soft palate and uvula should move upward together. The patient should also be able to feel the light touch of a swab on the posterior third of the tongue.

To check the vagus nerve, put your hand on the patient's throat and ask him to swallow. If the swallowing reflex is intact, check the patient's gag reflex by touching a cotton swab to the back of the throat.

8. Spinal accessory nerve (XI)

This nerve controls the sternocleidomastoid and trapezius muscles of the neck.

The sternocleidomastoid muscle is tested by placing your hand on the side of the patient's chin and asking him to push against the resistance of your hand (Figure 3-3). Note any atrophy, spasms, or weakness, and then repeat the procedure on the other side of the chin.

Figure 3-3 *Assessing spinal accessory nerve (cranial nerve XI) function*

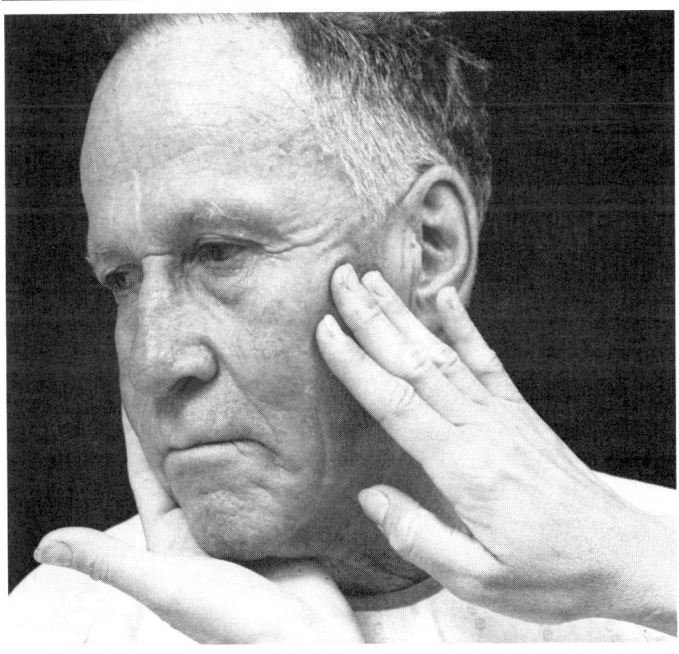

Evaluate the strength of the trapezius muscles by having the patient shrug his shoulders as you press down on them. Note any asymmetry or difficulty in movement.

9. Hypoglossal nerve (XII)

This nerve regulates all tongue movements, and is tested by asking the patient to push his tongue laterally against a tongue depressor. Inspect the tongue for any deviations, atrophy, or tremors.

F. Cerebellar function

The cerebellum controls balance and coordination, and a number of tests are performed to evaluate its functioning. In the tests that follow, observe the patient's ability to carry out all actions accurately and smoothly.

1. Begin the first test by having the patient sit with his eyes open and arms outstretched. Ask him to touch his finger to his nose, first with one hand, then with the other. Ask him to repeat the task with his eyes closed.
2. Next, with his eyes open, ask the patient to touch his nose and then touch your finger in rapid succession. Change the position of your finger as he continues to do this. Repeat this test with the other hand.
3. With the patient sitting, ask him to pat his knees alternately with his palms and the backs of his hands. Next, ask the patient to touch his fingers rapidly with the thumb of the same hand. Repeat with his other hand.
4. With the patient lying on his back, ask him to move his heel down the shin of his opposite leg, first with one foot, then with the other. Then ask the patient to draw a figure 8 in the air with each foot.
5. In the last test, with the patient barefoot, ask him to stand with his feet together, first with his eyes open and then with them closed (Romberg's test). Ask the patient to walk naturally with his eyes open, and then closed. Finally, ask the patient to walk in a heel-to-toe pattern. Be sure to stand near him so you can support him in case he starts to fall.

G. Sensory evaluation

Evaluation of the sensory system determines the patient's ability to perceive different sensations *with his eyes closed*. Compare the sensations on the two sides of the body, and in the distal and proximal parts of each extremity. Also, determine the extent of the sensory changes (e.g., unilateral, bilateral, or confined to one area).

1. Testing for primary sensations

a. Superficial tactile sensation. With a piece of cotton, stroke the patient's hands, arms, trunk, legs, and feet. Switch from one side of the body back to the other and compare the sensitivity of the distal and proximal parts.

b. Superficial pain. Follow the above procedure using a pin or other pointed instrument.

c. Sensitivity to temperature. Touch the patient's body with test tubes of hot and cold water. Ask the patient to tell you what he feels.

d. Sensitivity to vibration. Place a vibrating tuning fork on various bony prominences: knuckle, wrist, elbow, shoulder, hip, knee, shin, and ankle. Ask the patient to tell you when the vibration stops.

e. Deep pressure/pain. To elicit a response, squeeze the Achilles tendons, calf, and forearm.

f. Sense of position. As you move the patient's fingers and toes, ask him if the digit is held up or down.

2. Tests to determine discriminatory sensation

a. Two-point discrimination. Simultaneously touch various parts of the patient's body with two sharp objects to determine whether the patient feels one or two pricks. Note the distance at which he can distinguish each point separately. The ability to perceive distance is more precise on the fingertips and toes than on more proximal points of the extremities.

b. Point discrimination. With the patient's eyes still closed, touch him with your finger, and ask him to point to where he was touched.

c. Recognition of shape and form (stereognostic function). Again with his eyes closed, ask the patient to identify familiar objects placed in his hand.

d. Texture discrimination. Ask the patient to identify material of various textures, such as wool, velvet, or cotton.

e. Graphesthesia (number identification). With a blunt instrument, draw a large number on the patient's palm, and ask him to identify it. Repeat the test on his other hand, using different numbers or letters.

f. Extinction phenomenon. Touch two identical areas on opposite sides of the body. The patient should feel both stimuli.

H. Motor function

The next step in the neurologic assessment is evaluation of motor function. This includes observing the patient's gait, noting any involuntary movements, and evaluating his muscle size, muscle tone, and muscle strength.

1. Gait

Ask the patient to walk back and forth. Observe his posture, position of face and head, arm swing, and leg movements. Note steadiness, stance, and position of legs. Following are the more common types of gait abnormalities that may indicate neurologic problems.

a. Spastic hemiparesis. The arm on the affected side is flexed against the body; the leg moves stiffly outward in a semicircle. There may be toe dragging. This condition is associated with unilateral, upper motor neuron disease, such as stroke.

b. Scissors gait. Steps are short, and the knees cross each other with each step. A scissors gait is found in paresis of the legs (e.g., multiple sclerosis).

c. Steppage gait. Feet are lifted high and brought down hard. Steppage gait is associated with lower motor neuron disease at the spinal cord level.

d. Ataxia. The gait is unsteady, lurching, and wide-based. The patient watches the ground to guide his steps, and cannot stand steadily with his feet together. Ataxia may be due to disease of the cerebellum or associated tracts, or loss of position sense in the legs.

e. Parkinsonian gait. The posture is stooped with hips, knees, and elbows slightly flexed. Steps are short and shuffling, with stiffness of movement. This gait is associated with the basal ganglionic defects of Parkinson's disease.

2. Involuntary movements

a. Tremors. These are rhythmic, back-and-forth trembling movements. *Intentional tremors* occur with voluntary movement and are a sign of cerebellar disorders. *Resting tremors* diminish with voluntary effort, and are often seen in Parkinson's disease.

b. Chorea. Chorea is rapid, sudden, jerky movements that can involve the limbs, trunk, or face. The movements are nonrepetitive and can be quite strong.

c. Athetosis. These slow, repetitive, writhing, and twisting movements, primarily of posture, may occur with cerebral palsy.

d. Tics. Tics are repetitive twitching of a muscle group, producing movements such as grimaces, winks, or shrugging of the shoulders. They may be neurologic or emotional in origin.

3. Muscle size

Inspect the patient for symmetry of the muscles, comparing both sides of his body. You may find it helpful to measure the circumference of his limbs with a tape measure to confirm the presence of atrophy.

4. Muscle tone

With the patient relaxed, palpate the muscles at rest and during passive range of motion exercises. Begin at the fingers, then move to the wrist, elbow, and shoulder, and move down to the ankle, knee, and hip. Compare his right side with his left and observe for any abnormalities of tone:
- Spasticity – resistance of the muscles to passive changes in position
- Rigidity – undue resistance of the muscles to movement in all directions
- Flaccidity – decreased muscle tone; weak, flabby muscle
- Pain on movement
- Cogwheel motion – jerking movements of the limbs.

5. Muscle strength

This is evaluated by putting the muscles of the major joints through a passive range of motion and then testing the strength of the muscles against gravity and against active resistance. Remember to compare corresponding muscles on both sides. Test muscle strength in the lower extremities with the patient lying on his back.

a. Upper arm strength. Ask the patient to close his eyes and extend his arms straight out, palms up, for 20 to 30 seconds. Observe for downward drifting or pronation of the palms on one side, which could suggest mild hemiparesis (paralysis affecting only one side of the body). Ask the patient to resist your attempt to push down each outstretched arm.

b. Shoulder strength. With his eyes closed, have the patient raise his arms over his head, with palms forward, for 20 to 30 seconds. Observe for downward drift, and again attempt to depress the patient's arms against his resistance.

c. Elbow strength. Attempt to straighten the patient's flexed elbow by depressing his wrist. Repeat this test with the other arm.

d. Wrist. With the patient's fisted hands flexed upward, try to pull them downward as the patient resists.

e. Grip. Place your index and middle fingers in the patient's hands, and ask him to squeeze as hard as possible as you try to pull your fingers from his grip.

f. Fingers. Ask the patient to spread his fingers (excluding the thumb), while you try to force them together. Then ask the patient to make a fist, and try to insert your thumb into it. It should not be easily done.

g. Hip flexion. Ask the patient to raise his thigh against your resistance.

h. Hip extension. Ask the patient to do shallow knee bends, first on one leg, then on the other. Or you may assess extension as the patient rises from a squatting position or climbs steps.

i. Hip abduction. Place your hands on the outsides of the patient's knees and ask him to spread his legs against your resistance.

j. Hip adduction. Ask the patient to hold his legs slightly apart and then bring them together as you place resistance on the insides of his knees.

k. Knee flexion. Ask the patient to bend his knee while keeping his foot on the bed. Try to straighten the leg against the patient's resistance, and repeat with the other leg.

l. Knee extension. Ask him to bend his knee with his foot resting on the bed. Ask him to straighten his leg against your resistance.

m. Plantar flexion of foot. Place your hand on the ball of the patient's foot and ask him to press down against it as you press up. Or ask the patient to walk on his toes.

n. Dorsiflexion of foot. Place your hand on top of his toes and ask the patient to pull his feet against your hand. Alternatively, you may ask the patient to walk on his heels.

I. Evaluation of reflexes

Testing the reflexes is an important part of the neurologic exam. Alterations in reflexes could indicate problems within the corticospinal tract (upper motor neuron disease), in the anterior horn cells or their axons (lower motor neuron disease), or in the sensory components of the muscles. There are three types of reflexes: deep tendon reflexes, superficial reflexes, and pathologic reflexes.

1. Deep tendon reflexes

Assess the deep tendon reflexes by briskly tapping the bony prominence or tendon with a reflex hammer. Normally, the muscle should respond with a sudden stretch and contraction. A 4+ reflex is very brisk; lack of response is graded zero. A 2+ reflex is normal.

a. Technique. The patient must be relaxed, with the extremities held in a flexed or semiflexed position. Hold the hammer loosely and tap using wrist rather than arm action. If you have difficulty eliciting a response, use a reinforcement technique: When examining the upper extremities,

Figure 3-4 *Testing the biceps reflex*

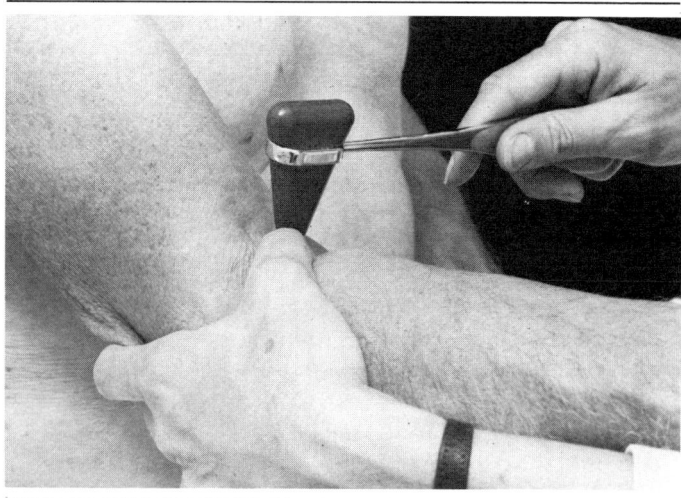

have the patient clench his teeth; when the lower extremities, have him lock his fingers together and pull. Always document your use of reinforcement. If you consistently find it hard to elicit deep tendon reflexes, check your technique.

b. Biceps reflex. With the patient sitting, his arms slightly flexed and palms down, place your thumb on the biceps tendon. Strike your thumb with the pointed end of the reflex hammer (Figure 3-4). You'll feel the contraction of the biceps and see a slight flexion at the elbow.

c. Triceps reflex. You can use either one of the following two methods: (1) Flex the patient's arm at the elbow and pull slightly across the chest, supporting his wrist with your hand. Strike the triceps tendon just above the elbow (Figure 3-5). You will see elbow extension and triceps muscle contraction. (2) Extend the patient's arm at a right angle to the body with forearm dangling and relaxed. Support under elbow with your hand and strike tendon with reflex hammer. Response will be the same.

Figure 3-5 *Testing the triceps reflex*

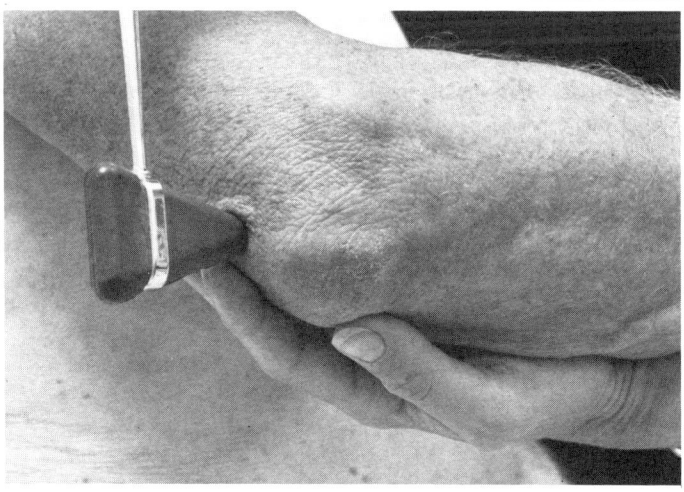

Figure 3-6 *Testing the supinator reflex*

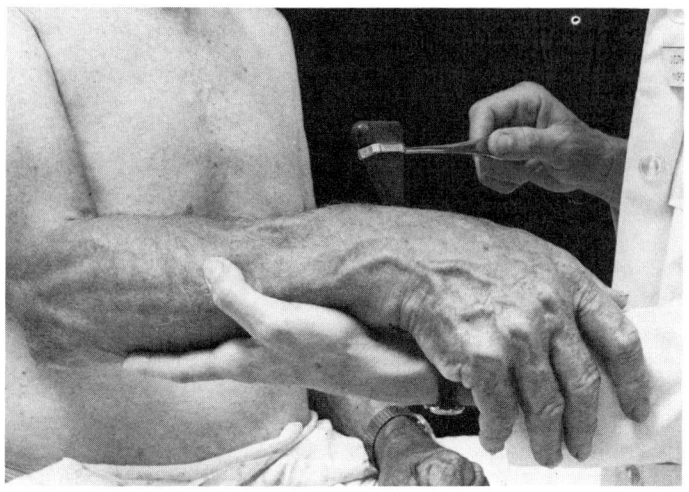

d. Brachioradialis reflex (supinator reflex). With the forearm resting on the patient's lap (or abdomen if the patient is lying down), palm down, strike the forearm just above the styloid process of the radius (Figure 3-6) and observe for flexion of the elbow and supination of the forearm.

e. Patellar reflex. As the patient sits with his knees flexed and feet hanging freely, tap the patellar tendon. Observe for contraction of the quadriceps with extension of the knee.

f. Achilles reflex. With the patient's feet hanging freely, pull the foot gently upward and tap above the heel with the blunt end of the hammer (Figure 3-7). The normal response is plantar flexion at the ankle.

Try to elicit ankle clonus—abnormal continued, rapid flexion and extension of the feet—by suddenly dorsiflexing the foot and applying sustained, moderate pressure.

2. Superficial reflexes

These are tested by lightly stroking the skin with a tongue blade or similar object.

Figure 3-7 *Testing the Achilles tendon reflex*

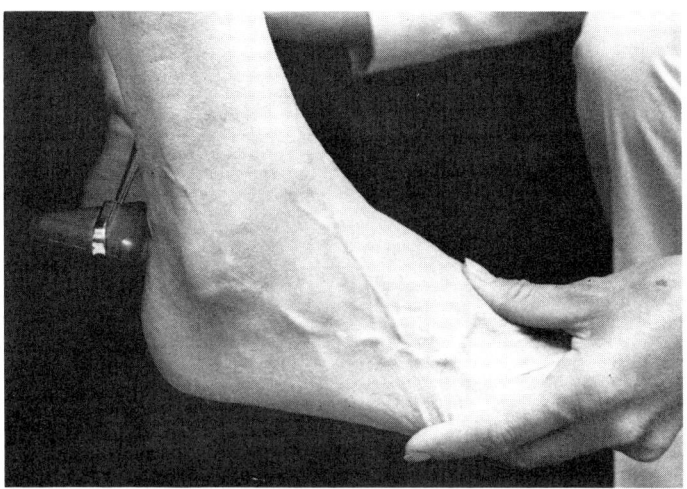

a. Abdominal reflex. Stroke the upper, middle, and lower abdomen. The abdominal muscles should contract, with retraction of the umbilicus toward the stimulated side.

b. Cremasteric reflex (in the male). Stroke the inner aspect of the upper leg. Normally, the testicle on the side being stroked will retract.

c. Plantar reflex. Begin by stroking the lateral aspect of the sole of the foot from heel to toe. Then direct the stimulus across the ball of the foot toward the medial aspect. The normal response is plantar flexion of the toes.

3. Pathologic reflexes

A positive response to the following tests is extension or dorsiflexion of the big toe, with fanning of the smaller toes (Figure 3-8). If present, this response indicates pyramidal tract disease.

a. Babinski. Attempt to elicit a plantar reflex.

b. Chaddock. Stroke under the lateral malleolus and along the lateral aspect of the dorsum of the foot.

Figure 3-8 *Pathologic reflex (Babinski)*

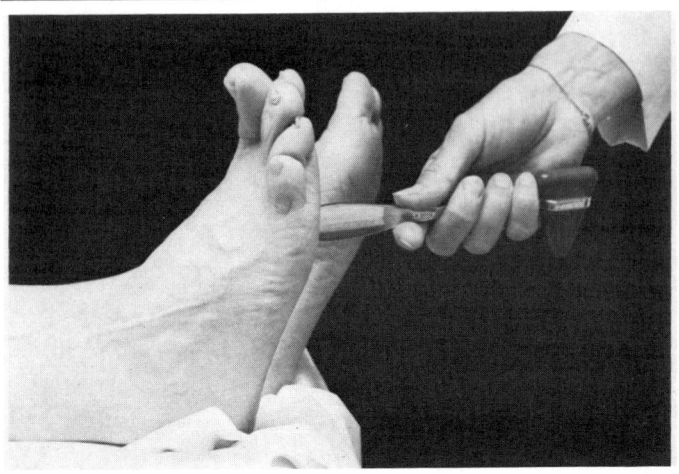

c. Oppenheim. With your thumb and index finger, press firmly on the anteromedian surface of the upper third of the tibia, and stroke toward the patient's ankle.

d. Gordon. Firmly squeeze the patient's calf muscle.

QUIZ

1. During the interview, general observations should be made regarding your patient's _____ and _____.

2. List the three areas in which orientation is tested:

3. List the four types of agnosia that could result from damage to the cerebral cortex:

4. The ability to carry out a skilled act requires _____ and _____.

5. Which of the following is a test for receptive aphasia?
   a. Ask the patient to answer a question.
   b. Ask the patient to write his name.
   c. Ask the patient to follow a command.
   d. Ask the patient to tell you his address.

Match the cranial nerves with their corresponding test.

6. Olfactory nerve _____
7. Optic nerve _____
8. Oculomotor, trochlear, abducens nerves _____
9. Trigeminal nerve _____
10. Facial nerve _____
11. Acoustic nerve _____
12. Glossopharyngeal and vagus nerves _____
13. Spinal accessory nerve _____
14. Hypoglossal nerve _____

a. Test for facial asymmetry
b. Test for gag reflex
c. Test of sense of smell
d. Weber test
e. Test of vision
f. Test of trapezius muscle strength
g. Extraocular movement
h. Test strength of tongue
i. Test facial sensation

15. Which of the following tests evaluate coordination?
   a. Touching nose with finger
   b. Walking heel to toe
   c. Arm raising
   d. Rinne test

16. Which of the following tests evaluate the presence of primary sensations?
   a. Two-point discrimination
   b. Sensitivity to vibration
   c. Testing for position sense
   d. Stereognostic function

17. Gait associated with unilateral, upper motor neuron disease is _____.

18. Slow, writhing, twisting movements are called _____.

19. If you have difficulty obtaining a reflex in your patient, you would:
   a. Recheck your technique
   b. Assume the patient has none
   c. Assume the patient is nervous and try later
   d. Utilize reinforcement techniques

ANSWERS
  1. Behavior; appearance.
  2. Person, place, time.
  3. Visual, auditory, tactile, spatial.
  4. Memory; normal motor strength.
  5. c.
  6. c.
  7. e.
  8. g.
  9. i.
  10. a.
  11. d.
  12. b.
  13. f.
  14. h.
  15. a, b.
  16. b, c.
  17. Spastic hemiparesis.
  18. Athetosis.
  19. a, d.

CHAPTER

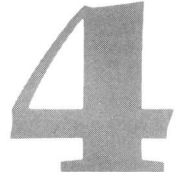

Alterations in Consciousness and Increased Intracranial Pressure

OBJECTIVES

After completing this chapter, you will be able to:

1. Describe the physiology of consciousness
2. Assess the patient with an alteration in consciousness
3. Utilize the Glasgow coma scale
4. Discuss the dynamics of intracranial pressure
5. Identify the signs and symptoms of increased intracranial pressure
6. Discuss factors that affect intracranial pressure
7. Identify the goals of medical and nursing management of the patient with increased intracranial pressure.

A. Etiology of changes in consciousness

Coma is the result of a dysfunction that has affected cerebral metabolism. It can be due to primary brain injury or disease or to systemic diseases that affect the brain secondarily. Examples of the former include vascular diseases such as ruptured aneurysm, thrombosis, embolism, or hemorrhage; trauma, which includes concussion, contusion, intracerebral hemorrhage, subdural hematoma, or epidural hematoma; lesions of the brain such as tumor or abscess; infections such as meningitis or encephalitis; and seizures. Systemic problems that can cause coma include uremia, hypoglycemia, diabetic ketoacidosis, hypertensive encephalopathy, drug overdose, heavy metal poisoning, alcohol, hypothermia, and carbon monoxide poisoning.

B. Physiology of consciousness

A conscious person responds fully to stimuli and indicates by his behavior and speech that he is aware of himself and his environment. Consciousness has two components: arousal, which is dependent on structures in the brain stem, and cognition, which includes functions controlled by the cerebral hemispheres.

Alterations in consciousness can range from mild stupor to severe coma. Coma may result from any dysfunction of the reticular activating system, from the brain stem to the cortex.

C. Assessing for alterations in consciousness

1. Levels of consciousness

The level of consciousness is one of the most important indicators of neurologic change, since an alteration is an early sign of brain dysfunction.

Auditory and painful stimuli are used to evaluate levels of consciousness. Minimal auditory stimulus (speaking to the patient) is used first, with progression of stimuli until a response is obtained. Painful stimuli are reserved for unconscious patients.

a. Terms that describe levels of consciousness. Labeling of levels of consciousness should be avoided, because uniform definitions are not available. Instead, describe the patient's behavior and his response to stimuli.
- Awake, alert – oriented to time, person, and place; short- and long-term memory intact; easily aroused; understands written and spoken words
- Alert with memory lapses – disoriented to time; poor attention span
- Drowsy and confused – disoriented to time and place and may gradually become disoriented to person; memory poor; lethargic; has difficulty responding to commands; may become agitated, particularly at night
- Delirium – restless, disoriented, agitated, and may hallucinate
- Stupor – very drowsy and generally unresponsive; aroused by repeated stimuli; withdraws purposefully from painful stimuli such as pressure on fingernails
- Coma – unarousable even with painful stimuli. In a deep coma the patient also lacks corneal, pupillary, and pharyngeal reflexes.

b. The Glasgow coma scale (GCS). The Glasgow coma scale (Figure 4-1) was designed to standardize observations for objective assessment of the level of consciousness. The scale is divided into three areas: eye opening, best motor response, and best verbal response. A numerical rating is given for each area, and the sum of all three areas is the final score. The highest score, 15, indicates a patient who is awake, oriented, and obeying commands. The lowest score, 3, indicates deep coma. A score of 7 or below is considered the level for coma.

2. Pupillary reactions

Assess the size and equality of the pupils, and their reaction to light: brisk, moderate, sluggish, or fixed (see Chapter 3). Abnormal responses and their meanings include:

a. Unilaterally dilated and unreactive pupil. This is usually due to compression of the oculomotor nerve by herniation of the temporal lobe. It may result from increased intra-

Figure 4-1 *The Glasgow coma scale*

Eyes	Open	Spontaneously	4
		To verbal command	3
		To pain	2
	No response		1
Best motor response	To verbal command	Obeys	6
	To painful stimulus*	Localizes pain	5
		Flexion-withdrawal	4
		Flexion-abnormal (decorticate rigidity)	3
		Extension (decerebrate rigidity)	2
		No response	1
Best verbal response†		Oriented and converses	5
		Disoriented and converses	4
		Inappropriate words	3
		Incomprehensible sounds	2
		No response	1
Total			3-15

*Apply knuckle to sternum, observe arms.
†Arouse patient with painful stimulus if necessary.

From Teasdale G, Jennett B: Assessment of coma and impaired consciousness: A practical scale. *Lancet* 2:81, 1974.

cranial pressure. If a new finding, it should be reported immediately to the physician.

b. Midposition (3 to 5 mm) nonreactive pupils. This finding is associated with midbrain damage or transtentorial herniation.

c. Small, unreactive pupils. Small, unreactive pupils usually result from pontine damage, and are also found with opiate drug overdoses.

d. One pupil smaller, both react to light. Hypothalamic damage due to transtentorial herniation produces this finding.

e. Dilated, unreactive pupils. These are usually found in terminal stages of illness, and are due to anoxia and ischemia. They may also be caused by atropine-like drugs. Emergency action is needed to prevent death.

3. Eye movement

In responsible patients, extraocular movements should be assessed. In the comatose patient, eye movement is absent, or the eyes move from side to side. The most useful test in comatose patients is the oculocephalic response, or doll's eyes maneuver. Briskly rotate the patient's head from side to side; normally the eyes will move in the direction opposite the rotating head. The reflex is absent when the eyes do not move and therefore follow the head movement. An abnormal response is due to a destructive lesion at the pontine-midbrain level. Barbiturate poisoning may also abolish the reflex.

4. Respiratory patterns

The respiratory pattern is helpful in localizing a possible lesion, and may occasionally determine the nature of the process.

a. Cheyne-Stokes respiration. Breathing alternates rhythmically between hyperventilation and apnea. This pattern usually indicates bilateral deep hemispheric and basal ganglionic dysfunction, but may also be caused by metabolic disorders such as diabetic coma and uremia.

b. Central neurogenic hyperventilation. These continual, rapid, regular respirations, with a rate of about 25/minute, cannot be attributed to hypoxemia if the arterial blood oxygen has been 70 mm Hg or greater for 24 hours. This condition is due to a lesion in the midbrain or pons.

c. Apneustic breathing. A prolonged inspiratory phase is followed by a pause that lasts 2 to 3 seconds. This pattern suggests lower pontine damage.

d. Cluster breathing. Clusters of irregular breathing are followed by periods of apnea at irregular intervals. The lesion is in the area of the upper medulla and lower pons.

e. Ataxic breathing. This consists of chaotic respirations with random deep and shallow breaths and pauses. It indicates damage to the medullary respiratory centers and carries a poor prognosis.

5. Pulse

Note the rate, rhythm, and quality of the pulse, and record whether it has been derived apically or radially. Bradycardia with a bounding pulse may be present in the later stages of increased intracranial pressure. Tachycardia may be indicative of poor cerebral oxygenation, internal bleeding, or the terminal stage of illness. Cardiac arrhythmias are not uncommon, especially if the cerebrospinal fluid contains blood or if the patient has undergone posterior fossa surgery.

6. Blood pressure

After taking the patient's blood pressure, compare the current findings with previous records to identify any changes or trends. Elevated pressure is a late sign of increased intracranial pressure. However, the blood pressure may also rise in response to a stimulus, such as suctioning, so evaluate all pertinent data. Low blood pressure indicates inadequate cerebral perfusion and neurologic deterioration.

7. Temperature

Elevations in temperature could be due to infection, either inside or outside the central nervous system, or to damage or compression of the hypothalamus, which regulates temperature. Hypothermia can result from the comatose state, spinal shock, or hypothalamic damage.

8. Sensory function

To evaluate sensory function in a patient with altered consciousness, apply a painful stimulus by pressing on a nail bed with the side of a pencil.

9. Motor function

If the patient is conscious, evaluate his ability to move all his extremities, as well as muscle strength. Compare the right and left sides.

If the patient is unconscious, you can assess motor function in two ways. First, lift both arms and release them; a paralyzed limb will fall more rapidly. Also test the legs. Next, apply a painful stimulus to each limb. If the motor tract is intact, the patient will withdraw the limb.

10. Abnormal posturing

Abnormal posturing is always evidence of motor damage.

a. Decorticate posturing. The arms, wrists, and fingers are flexed, with adduction of the arms and extension and internal rotation of the legs. Decorticate posturing occurs with lesions in the area of the pons, including the internal capsule, basal ganglia, and thalamus.

b. Decerebrate posturing. In its severe form, decerebrate posturing includes opisthotonus with clenched teeth, arms extended and hyperpronated, and legs extended with feet in a plantar-flexed position. Decerebration is a sign of more severe dysfunction than decortication. Decerebrate and decorticate posturing may alternate, or one side may be decerebrate and one side decorticate.

11. Reflexes

Abnormal reflexes may also be present. A positive Babinski reflex (see Figure 3-15) indicates pressure on the pyramidal tract. The grasp reflex indicates massive bilateral cerebral dysfunction. Here, the patient grasps and holds on to the source of a stimulus when the palm is stroked.

D. Dynamics of intracranial pressure

Basic to understanding intracranial pressure is the Monro-Kellie hypothesis. According to this hypothesis, the brain, cerebrospinal fluid, and cerebral blood vessels fill the rigid skull. An increase in any one of these three must be compensated for by a decrease in one or both of the others, or intracranial pressure will rise. Cerebrospinal fluid is the most easily and rapidly displaced.

The amount of displacement of any of the components is limited; after a certain level of homeostasis has been reached, decompensation with increased intracranial pressure results.

Normal intracranial pressure is a level between 80 and 180 mm of water, or 0 to 15 mm of Hg. Intracranial pressure above 15 mm Hg (200 mm water pressure) is considered abnormally high.

E. Alterations in intracranial pressure

1. Disturbances due to increased brain mass

An increase in brain tissue volume can be caused by a tumor, abscess, hematoma, or cerebral edema. As the volume of tissue expands, it is displaced downward through the tentorial opening and foramen magnum, where it compresses the brain stem. This results in coma, respiratory alterations, and, eventually, death.

2. Alteration of cerebrospinal fluid circulation or absorption

Blockage or overproduction of cerebrospinal fluid can cause an overaccumulation of fluid, or hydrocephalus. This increases the size of the ventricles and exerts pressure on surrounding brain tissue. Eventually, this pressure causes atrophy of the cerebral white matter.

3. Alterations in blood volume autoregulation

Cerebral blood flow is automatically regulated by changes in the diameter of blood vessels within the brain. For example, an increase in carbon dioxide in the blood (hypercapnia) causes vasodilation, thereby increasing blood volume in the brain, in order to maintain oxygenation. Conversely, a decreased carbon dioxide level in the blood causes vasoconstriction and decreases the blood volume.

Increases in intracranial pressure decrease cerebral blood flow. Normally, perfusion of the brain is maintained by arterial blood pressure that is greater than the intracranial pressure. If the intracranial pressure rises, the arterial pressure must also rise to maintain cerebral perfusion. However, this autoregulatory mechanism becomes impaired when intracranial pressure exceeds approximately 33 mm Hg.

F. Signs and symptoms of increased intracranial pressure

1. Decrease in the level of consciousness

This is usually a reliable indicator of deterioration, because the cells of the cerebral cortex are highly sensitive to the decreased oxygen supply that results from increased intracranial pressure. Lack of oxygen makes the patient drowsy or disoriented.

2. Pupillary changes

The pupils on the side of the lesion first constrict, then progressively dilate. The direct light response becomes sluggish, then nonreactive. Eventually, the deterioration progresses to the point where the pupils are fixed. This is caused by compression of the oculomotor nerve (cranial nerve III).

3. Changes in vital signs

Initially, systemic blood pressure increases in response to ischemia of the vasomotor center of the brain. As the patient's condition worsens, the decompensatory phase begins, causing the blood pressure to drop.

In the compensatory stage, the pulse falls to about 60/minute, and is described as bounding. With decompensation, the pulse then becomes rapid, irregular, and thready.

Alterations in the respiratory pattern depend on the extent of brain dysfunction. (Refer to section C4 earlier in this chapter.)

The patient's temperature is usually normal unless he has a systemic infection. In the decompensatory phase, however, the temperature is likely to be elevated to very high levels.

4. Motor and sensory dysfunction

Motor loss can progress from hemiparesis to hemiplegia. With further deterioration, signs of abnormal posturing are apparent. Sensory loss is also evident as the patient becomes less responsive to touch, pain, temperature, and proprioception.

5. Papilledema

Papilledema (see Chapter 3) is seen when intracranial pressure has become markedly elevated. It does not occur in all patients.

6. Headache

Although headache rarely occurs with increased intracranial pressure, its presence is due to dilation of vessels and stretching of arteries.

7. Vomiting

Vomiting is rare in increased intracranial pressure. When it does occur, it may come without nausea and be projectile.

G. Factors that affect intracranial pressure

1. Hypercapnia and hypoxemia

These factors can cause intracranial pressure to increase, because they cause vasodilation of cerebral vessels and increased blood volume. Frequent blood gas analysis is necessary to evaluate blood oxygenation.

2. Valsalva's maneuver

This causes an increase in intrathoracic pressure, which impedes venous return from the brain, thereby increasing intracranial pressure. Valsalva's maneuver can be initiated by changing position in bed or by straining at stool. To prevent the patient from initiating the maneuver, administer stool softeners, and tell him to exhale whenever he is being moved or turned in bed.

3. Coughing and sneezing

Like Valsalva's maneuver, coughing and sneezing cause an increase in intracranial pressure by impeding venous return from the brain. Take precautionary measures to control the patient's coughing or sneezing as much as possible.

4. Isometric exercises

Isometric exercises increase systemic blood pressure, thus increasing intracranial pressure. Such exercises are therefore contraindicated when intracranial pressure is increased.

Passive range of motion exercises do not produce this effect and can safely be a part of the patient's care.

5. Sleep

REM (rapid eye movement) sleep causes an increase in cerebral activity, which increases blood volume and, in turn, increases intracranial pressure. The REM stage of sleep cannot be prevented, so it's important to avoid measures, such as turning the patient, that exacerbate intracranial pressure when REM sleep does occur. REM sleep can be identified by fluttering of the eyes beneath the eyelids.

6. Position of the body

Positions such as severe angulation of the neck, extreme hip flexion, the prone position, and Trendelenburg's position all increase intracranial pressure and should be avoided.

7. Vasodilating drugs

Any drugs that increase the blood flow to the brain would raise already increased intracranial pressure.

H. Management of increased intracranial pressure

1. Medical management

The ultimate goal of medical management is elimination of the cause by either medical or surgical treatment. General principles include maintaining an airway for adequate ventilation, hyperventilation to promote cerebral vasoconstriction, and drug therapy with osmotic diuretics, corticosteroids (see Appendix), and anticonvulsants.

Hypothermia has been used to reduce the brain's need for nutrients. Drainage of cerebrospinal fluid from the ventricles through a catheter may temporarily control intracranial pressure.

In severe uncontrolled elevation of intracranial pressure, barbiturate coma may be used. Short-acting barbiturates are administered to induce coma, which promotes cerebral vasoconstriction and slows cerebral metabolism.

2. Nursing management

Nursing management focuses on preventing further increases in intracranial pressure. Care includes maintenance of ventilation, frequent neurologic assessment, proper positioning, monitoring fluids, administration of drugs, and general nursing measures demanded by the patient's condition. Chapter 5 discusses nursing interventions based on nursing diagnoses.

QUIZ

1. The two components of consciousness are _____ and _____.

2. Which of the following statements concerning the reticular activating system (RAS) is *not* true?
    a. Made up of fiber bundles that travel from the brain stem to the cerebral cortex
    b. Stimulation of the RAS causes coma
    c. Controls sleep and wakefulness
    d. Controls part of our ability to direct our attention

3. Which of the following stimuli are utilized to assess levels of consciousness?
    a. Auditory and painful stimuli
    b. Auditory and visual stimuli
    c. Visual and painful stimuli
    d. Auditory and light stimuli

4. You are assessing Mr. K's level of consciousness utilizing the Glasgow coma scale. What is his score if he opens his eyes in response to pain, flexes and withdraws but utters sounds that are not understandable?
   a. 9
   b. 5
   c. 8
   d. 10

5. Mr. K has suddenly developed a dilated and unreactive pupil on the right side. What would you do?
   a. Check it again in 10 minutes
   b. Chart your findings
   c. Call the physician immediately
   d. Administer oxygen, if ordered

6. Mr. K develops Cheyne-Stokes respiration. This respiratory pattern is an indication of dysfunction in what area of the brain?
   a. Pons
   b. Midbrain
   c. Medulla
   d. Deep in hemispheres and basal ganglion

7. Which of the following is *not* true of decerebrate posturing?
   a. Less severe sign than decorticate posturing
   b. May occur on only one side of the body
   c. Arms are extended and hyperpronated
   d. Feet are plantar-flexed

8. Which of the following is *not* true regarding the dynamics of intracranial pressure?
   a. An increase in brain mass will cause a decrease in the volume of cerebrospinal fluid
   b. Rapid increases in volume are better tolerated
   c. Small volume increases are better tolerated
   d. When skull contents cannot compensate for increasing volume, intracranial pressure increases

9. Signs and symptoms of increased intracranial pressure include:
   a. Decrease in level of consciousness
   b. Initial pupillary dilation then constriction
   c. Bradycardia and hypertension
   d. Motor and sensory loss

10. Hypercapnia and hypoxemia are serious if they occur with increased intracranial pressure since they cause:
   a. Dilation of cerebral vessels
   b. An increase in cerebral edema
   c. Constriction of cerebral vessels and ischemia
   d. A decrease in cerebral blood volume

ANSWERS
   1. Arousal; cognition.
   2. b.
   3. a.
   4. c.
   5. c.
   6. d.
   7. a.
   8. b.
   9. a, c, d.
10. a.

CHAPTER 5

Nursing Management of the Neurologic Patient

OBJECTIVES

After completing this chapter, you will be able to:

1. Identify the nursing management problems of the neurologic patient according to nursing diagnosis

2. Discuss the nursing management of the neurologic patient according to specific nursing diagnoses.

A. Introduction

Nursing management of the neurologic patient is a challenge that requires much knowledge and skill. The needs of the patient can be many, varied, and complex.

Following the first step in the nursing process, assessment, you should formulate a nursing diagnosis, plan care, and implement that plan. This chapter discusses the needs and nursing management of the neurologic patient according to specific nursing diagnoses.

B. Impaired gas exchange

Many neurologic problems can impair gas exchange. Paralyzed or immobilized patients require intensive nursing measures to prevent respiratory embarrassment.

1. Maintaining an airway

Your first major goal is to maintain a patent airway. Unless this is contraindicated, position the patient on his side with his head slightly extended and with the head of the bed at a 30 degree angle. This position allows for drainage of secretions. Never place an unconscious patient on his back. Turn the patient at least every 2 hours to prevent pooling of secretions.

2. Pulmonary toilet

If the patient is cooperative, encourage him to breathe deeply and cough frequently. (**Remember:** Coughing is contraindicated with increased intracranial pressure.) If the patient is unable to do this, institute postural drainage, chest physiotherapy, and suctioning. In order to maintain a patent airway and suction effectively, an oral or nasal airway may be utilized.

3. Oxygen

Oxygen therapy may be used. To prevent drying of the nares, the oxygen must be humidified. Keep nasal passages moist and free of dried secretions by cleaning them with saline-moistened cotton applicators and lubricating them with mineral oil.

4. Tracheostomy care

Certain neurologic diseases, such as myasthenia gravis, Guillain-Barré syndrome, and stroke, often cause respiratory impairment. Have a tracheostomy set nearby for emergency use. Mechanical ventilation may become necessary.

Patients whose airway is maintained by an endotracheal or tracheostomy tube will require added nursing measures. Periodically hyperinflate the patient's lungs with an Ambu bag to prevent atelectasis and to loosen secretions. Instillation of several milliliters of sterile normal saline into the tube before suctioning will help promote coughing and increase lung expansion. Follow this by hyperinflation, and then suction for no more than 15 seconds to prevent hypercapnia.

Tracheostomy care with aseptic technique at least every 4 hours is necessary. Follow your hospital's procedure.

The patient requiring a mechanical ventilator will require added nursing measures; however, these specialized procedures are beyond the scope of this book.

C. Alteration in tissue perfusion

Depending on the neurologic condition, cardiac function and circulation may be affected. Nursing management should be directed toward maintaining normal circulation with prevention of stasis and clotting of blood.

1. Mobilization

The first step in achieving this goal is to keep the patient as mobile as possible through the use of ambulation, frequent position changes, and active and passive exercises.

2. Positioning

If the patient can't move himself, use pillows, rolls, and other devices to position him in good body alignment. Do not allow paralyzed limbs to dangle, since edema may develop.

3. Preventing thrombophlebitis

Use elastic or support hose to prevent thrombophlebitis. Be sure the stockings aren't too tight. Remove them several times a day to inspect the patient's legs and for bathing. Low-dose heparin or aspirin may also be ordered to prevent thrombophlebitis.

4. Maintaining cerebral blood flow

Orthostatic hypotension is a common result of prolonged bed rest and a side effect of several neurologic drugs. Avoid sudden position changes in a patient who is susceptible. Gradual raising of the head while monitoring blood pressure and pulse is necessary. For a paralyzed patient, a tilt table may be used.

A patient with compromised cerebral blood flow, as in the acute phase following stroke, should have his head placed in a level position.

5. Cardiac monitoring

The presence of cardiac arrhythmias may require cardiac monitoring and specific drug therapy. Hypertension may be due to a pre-existing problem or cerebral decompensation. The cause must be treated.

D. Impaired physical mobility

An alteration of mobility due to a neurologic disease can range from mild weakness to severe paralysis. Rigidity and spasticity also affect mobility. The unconscious patient also requires nursing care directed toward maintaining musculoskeletal function and preventing orthopedic disabilities.

Maintaining mobility is the primary method of preventing musculoskeletal complications. Proper positioning in bed and chair along with active and passive range of motion exercises is important.

1. Maintaining proper body alignment

Proper body alignment can be maintained by pillows, rolls, and footboards. Splints and slings are helpful in maintaining an extremity or part of an extremity in a functional position. Remove splints every 4 hours to check for skin irritation and to perform exercises. High-top sneakers can be worn to prevent footdrop, but remove them periodically. Avoid long intervals of sitting in a bed or chair or positions with hips and knees flexed.

2. Range of motion exercises

Spasticity, which can occur with paraplegia and quadriplegia, can best be prevented and treated by passive range of motion. However, rigidity, as in Parkinson's disease (see Chapter 10), can be worsened by stimulation. Exercises should be done slowly, with proper support of joints.

3. Traction

Patients requiring orthopedic traction also require specialized care. Be sure that traction is secure at all times and that proper body alignment is maintained. Meticulous care is necessary for pin and tong sites. Examine entrance sites regularly for evidence of infection. Usually the area is cleaned with hydrogen peroxide and antiseptic ointment is applied. Skin care is especially important for patients in traction.

E. Impairment of skin integrity

Patients who are immobile are at great risk for skin breakdown. Meticulous nursing care is the most effective preventive measure.

1. Skin care

Keep the patient's skin clean and dry, lubricating as necessary. Turn the patient every 1 to 2 hours and massage reddened areas and bony prominences. Examine areas such as the ears, head, heels, and ankles for irritation and protect these areas from pressure. A turning schedule posted above the patient's bed will be a reminder to all concerned with the patient's care. Give back care every 4 hours. Maintain proper positioning in bed, avoiding contact between skin surfaces or pressure of one body part on another.

Utilize a turning sheet to move the patient and provide proper support for him when he's sitting in the bed or chair. Sliding downwards exerts a shearing force on the skin — a primary factor in decubitus formation. Air or foam mattresses, specialized beds, and foam heel and elbow pads will also help prevent skin breakdown.

2. Care of incontinent patients

Immediately clean an incontinent patient. Avoid the use of plastic incontinence pads, since they negate the advantages of any specialized mattresses and can cause skin irritation if they become wrinkled or wet.

A patient on a hypothermia blanket may perspire profusely and require additional care to keep him dry. A bath blanket used as a sheet may help absorb some of the perspiration, but change it frequently.

F. Self-care deficit (hygiene)

Many patients with neurologic disease are unable to meet some or all of their basic hygienic needs.

1. Bathing and shampooing

The patient may require partial or total help with his bath. Take this opportunity to turn the patient, inspect and massage his skin, and provide range of motion exercise. Male patients should be shaved.

Keep your patient's hair neatly combed. Wash hair as needed according to hospital procedure.

2. Mouth care

Give mouth care every 3 to 4 hours. Cooperative patients require toothbrushing and a mouth rinse. A patient with altered consciousness can have his teeth brushed and his mouth suctioned with a catheter. Irrigate the patient's mouth by placing his head to the side and instilling a solution of 3 parts mouthwash and 1 part peroxide with a syringe while applying continuous oral suction. Lubricate the lips with petroleum jelly.

3. Eye care

If the corneal reflex (Chapter 3) is diminished or absent, special eye care is necessary to prevent corneal abrasions. Remove dried secretions with sterile cotton balls moistened with sterile saline. Sterile saline or artificial tears should be instilled in the eye every 4 hours. If a comatose patient's eyes will not shut properly, they should be covered with eye shields or taped closed. Occasionally antibiotic eye ointment is ordered to prevent infection.

For the patient who develops periocular edema and ecchymosis following trauma or craniotomy, warm and cold compresses can be alternated to reduce edema.

4. Nail care

Fingernails and toenails should be kept clean and clipped as necessary. It may be helpful to soak the patient's hands and feet in warm water prior to doing this.

G. Alteration in fluid volume

The neurologic patient may need to receive fluids intravenously because of decreased level of consciousness, nausea, dysphagia, or absence of bowel sounds, or to provide a route for intravenous medications. If so, fluid intake and output and body weight should be monitored daily. In acute situations, measure urinary output every hour.

Fluid restriction — oral and intravenous — is often ordered if cerebral edema is present or could possibly occur, in an attempt to prevent an increase in intracranial pressure. But if there's no danger of cerebral edema, fluids should be encouraged in situations where mobility is decreased.

Diabetes insipidus, due to inadequate antidiuretic hormone secretion by the pituitary, can occur after cranial surgery, especially if the pituitary is involved. The patient will produce large amounts of urine with low specific gravity and can rapidly become dehydrated. Nursing responsibilities include accurate measurement of intake and output and specific gravity (1.005 or less is a low reading). In this situation, oral fluids are forced or intravenous fluids are adjusted. Diabetes insipidus is usually temporary.

H. Alteration in nutrition

Here, your goal should be prevention or reversal of excessive weight loss and protein breakdown in the body.

Patients with neurologic problems may have decreased appetite, difficulty in swallowing ability, and diminished peristalsis. Alterations in consciousness also affect the ability to maintain adequate nutrition. Increased metabolic need, prolonged bed rest, and maintenance on intravenous fluids all contribute to tissue breakdown.

1. Meeting nutritional needs

On admission, the patient should be weighed to establish a baseline. A patient who can eat should be encouraged to maintain an adequate intake. If appetite is poor, several small meals could replace three large ones. Encourage foods high in protein and calories. Consult the dietitian to help meet patients' special needs and preferences. Making mealtimes social events is often helpful.

If weakness is preventing the patient from finishing a meal, offer assistance. Patients who have difficulty chewing may need a soft diet. Nutritional supplements may help meet the patient's needs.

2. Special needs of the myasthenic patient

A myasthenic patient needs to be encouraged to eat slowly. Giving him his medications 45 minutes prior to meals may increase his strength. Have suction equipment available to prevent aspiration.

3. Dealing with dysphagia

Patients with potential dysphagia, as well as those who have experienced it, need to be evaluated before each meal for their ability to swallow. Do this by observing the ability to swallow a sip of water. A speech therapist may be consulted and a feeding program designed. Feeding is best done in the upright position with torso forward and head flexed, since bowing the head aids the swallowing effort.

Liquids are most difficult to swallow. Milk products form excessive mucus and are not good choices. Avoid foods that require chewing, like meats. Semisolids are easiest to swallow because they hold their shape. Some patients may take time to regain swallowing function or may never do so, and should be fed via nasogastric or gastrostomy tube.

4. Tube feedings

An unconscious patient may initially be maintained on intravenous solutions with added potassium and vitamins. When peristalsis returns, as evidenced by bowel sounds and bowel movements, nasogastric feedings are begun. If enteral feeding is to be administered over the long term, a gastrostomy tube is inserted surgically. By either route, the patient is usually given commercially prepared liquid feedings either intermittently (every 3 to 4 hours) or continuously by gravity drip or pump.

a. Intermittent feedings. Before each intermittent feeding, elevate the patient's head 70 degrees to 90 degrees and aspirate stomach contents. The physician usually will specify the amount of aspirate (usually 70 to 100 ml) that contraindicates a feeding. Once feeding is begun, observe for signs of restlessness, cyanosis, and vomiting. Afterward, flush tube with water and keep patient upright for 1 hour.

b. Continuous feeding. If the patient is receiving continuous feeding, check for tube placement and stomach contents every 4 hours. Maintain the head of the bed in at least a 45-degree angle and observe for signs of difficulty or intolerance.

c. Diarrhea. Some tube feeding solutions are highly concentrated and should be given with water to prevent dehydration. The occurrence of diarrhea may require stopping the feeding for a time or changing the type of solution.

5. Parenteral hyperalimentation

Parenteral hyperalimentation may be utilized temporarily if a patient has experienced excessive weight loss, sluggish peristalsis, nausea, or abdominal distention. This should be administered according to hospital procedure.

I. Alteration in bowel elimination

An alteration in bowel elimination in neurologic patients can be due to decreased mobility, inadequate diet, limitation of fluids, certain medications, or lack of sensation, sphincter control, and muscular ability to expel stool.

1. Constipation

The most common problem is constipation, which can lead to distention and fecal impaction. Monitor and record bowel movements. If normal, formed stools are absent, you should perform rectal exams periodically for stool.

To maintain normal elimination patterns, include roughage and juices in the diet, if possible. If this isn't contraindicated, increase fluid intake to 2,000 to 3,000 ml per day. Prophylactic stool softeners may be ordered.

For an unconscious patient, a bowel program that includes a stool softener and mild laxative should be started. Usually enemas are contraindicated, since they can elicit Valsalva's maneuver and increase intracranial pressure.

2. Bowel training

For patients who are unable to control bowel action, bowel training is necessary. Establish a time of day for a bowel movement, based on previous patterns, and use a suppository to help establish regular habits.

3. Diarrhea

Frequent liquid stools may indicate fecal impaction. This may be treated with stool softeners, suppositories, manual extraction or enemas, if not contraindicated.

Diarrhea is often associated with intolerance to a tube feeding formula or to certain drugs that affect the normal flora of the gastrointestinal tract. The cause of the diarrhea should be determined and treated.

J. Alteration in patterns of urinary elimination

In order to prevent problems of inadequate urine output, urinary stasis, renal calculi, and urinary tract infection, encourage and help the patient drink 2 to 3 liters of fluid a day, unless contraindicated. Divide this intake between the three nursing shifts to ensure it will be achieved.

1. Urine testing

Check urine for clarity, color, sediment, protein, blood, and glucose. To evaluate hydration, measure specific gravity, check serum electrolytes, and observe skin turgor.

2. Management of incontinence

Simple incontinence caused by an altered level of consciousness should be treated by good skin care and frequent linen changes. An external collecting device may be effective for male patients. Indwelling catheters should be avoided because of the danger of infection.

Patients with an intellectual deficit may fail to recognize the need to urinate. Try to identify voiding times and offer the opportunity to void beforehand. Some fluid restriction prior to bedtime may help prevent sleep incontinence. For men, again, external catheters can be used.

Some patients may have occasional accidental incontinence. It may be due to the urinal's being out of reach or trouble finding the nursing call light. Determine the cause and find a solution. Again, offer the opportunity to void frequently.

3. Intermittent catheterization

A patient with areflexic (atonic) bladder due to spinal cord or peripheral nerve damage or spinal shock has no voluntary control. This can result in bladder distention and overflow incontinence with constant, dribbling urine. Initially an indwelling catheter is used, but treatment should progress to intermittent catheterization on a regular schedule. The patient may be taught this technique.

4. Bladder training

If some sensation remains, as in partial cord lesions, cerebral trauma, stroke, brain tumor, or multiple sclerosis, the patient may be able to progress to scheduled bladder training. The method used depends on the individual patient. Manual pressure on the suprapubic area (Credé method), straining, or contracting abdominal muscles may assist in bladder evacuation. Initially, check residual urine immediately after voiding to determine the method's effectiveness.

5. Indwelling catheter care

The patient with an indwelling catheter should receive catheter care at least twice daily according to hospital procedure. To prevent infection, avoid disconnecting the tubing and drainage bag and raising the drainage bag above bladder level. Check the tubing for kinks.

K. Potential for injury

Patient safety is an important aspect of patient care. Use side rails, adequate lighting, and restraints when needed to help prevent accidents.

The confused or agitated patient requires an orderly, hazard-free environment with good lighting. Restraints may be needed for sitting in a bed or chair. Utilize chairs with detachable tables. Watch mobile patients who could wander away. Always keep beds in the low position.

For unconscious patients, the side rails of the bed should be elevated at all times. Use restraints only when a patient could harm himself. When restraints are used, be sure to check frequently for skin irritation, and remove them for range of motion exercise.

Neurologic dysfunction often causes seizures. Be sure to institute seizure safety precautions in those situations (see Chapter 6).

L. Alteration in comfort

If neurologic dysfunction causes pain, perform a thorough assessment before taking any pain relief measures. Nursing measures include administering pain medications, offering basic comfort techniques, and diversional activities. Heat can be applied to painful muscles.

Certain types of pain may be controlled by surgery or stimulation. Hypnosis, biofeedback, relaxation techniques, and operant conditioning may also be utilized.

M. Impaired communication

Impairment of communication may be neurologic in origin or due to interventions such as tracheostomy.

1. Total inability to speak

If the patient is unable to speak because of a tracheostomy, ask yes/no questions and supply paper and pencils. If the patient cannot move, as in Guillain-Barré syndrome, you'll need to use your ingenuity in addition to such aids as picture and alphabet boards. The patient may be able to communicate by blinking his eyes—for example, one blink for "yes," two blinks for "no."

2. Expressive aphasia

If the patient is experiencing expressive aphasia, use pictures or objects for communication. Speak clearly, in short phrases, and do not raise your voice. Point to objects and name them. Ask him to repeat sounds and words. Allow him time to speak, and avoid correcting errors. Encourage the patient to write, if possible, or use an alphabet board so he can spell out words. Anticipate his needs.

3. Receptive aphasia

Patients with receptive aphasia need a distraction-free environment. Speak slowly and do not raise your voice. Utilize gestures and repeat words and sentences as necessary. Use simple phrases with whatever words the patient understands.

4. Speech therapy referral

A speech therapist is invaluable in diagnosing communication dysfunctions and also in determining the method of management.

N. Sensory perceptual alteration

1. Visual

The extent of any visual defect must be determined. The visually impaired patient must be protected from injury and helped to gain independence.

A patient with severe visual dysfunction should have only necessary articles placed within reach. Always remember to orient him to the environment. Address the patient as you enter the room, and tell him your name. Tell him when you are leaving. Help him use other senses to gather information about his environment.

The patient with diplopia should have the affected eye patched or the lens of his eyeglasses occluded on the affected side.

Approach the patient with hemianopsia from the unaffected side. Encourage him to turn his head to compensate for the deficit.

2. Tactile

Patients who have lost tactile sensation have special needs. They must be taught to be vigilant and protect involved body parts from trauma, heat, cold, and pressure. They may need to check their skin routinely for signs of irritation or trauma. Bath water should be checked with an uninvolved body part or a thermometer.

O. Ineffective coping

The patient with a neurologic disorder may have difficulty emotionally coping with his disease and/or disabilities. Spend time with your patient to develop a relationship of trust. Encourage the patient to express his fears, anxieties, and concerns. Answer his questions and help find solutions to his problems.

1. The grieving process

The patient may go through a grieving process when he understands his loss of function is permanent or his disease is incurable. Initially, he may deny the disease or injury. This is a normal reaction and should be allowed. It is not healthy, however, for the patient to become fixed at the denial stage.

Following denial comes anger, which can lead to either despair or acceptance. The patient needs the hospital staff and family to help him see his personal worth. He needs support and encouragement to deal realistically with his altered lifestyle.

2. Supporting the family

The patient's family will also be affected by his injury or illness. The family may react by reorganizing and becoming stronger or it may resent the demands placed on it by the illness. You should support the family through this crisis by making members feel comfortable within a strange environment, explaining equipment, and helping them understand the patient's behavior.

Encourage family members to visit and assist with physical care when appropriate. Above all, keep the patient's relatives informed about the situation and help them express their fears and concerns.

P. Knowledge deficit

Patient education is a major part of your role. Help the patient understand his disease, the diagnostic studies he will undergo, and the treatments he will receive. Formulate an individual teaching plan that outlines all the patient's learning needs and methods to meet them. Be sure to include significant others in the teaching process.

Q. Rehabilitation

The rehabilitation process is individualized for each patient. All members of the health-care team, as well as the patient and family, should be involved in the planning and implementation of the program. The goal of rehabilitation is to help the patient become as independent as possible. He may need to be taught how to perform activities of daily living, transfers, and exercises. He may need to learn to walk again or develop new ways to communicate. The process is long and slow, and the patient needs your support and encouragement.

QUIZ

1. Maintenance of a patent airway includes:
   a. Positioning the patient on his side
   b. Positioning the patient on his back
   c. Flexing the patient's head
   d. Slightly extending the patient's head
   e. Maintaining the head of the bed at a 30-degree angle
2. Care of the patient with a tracheostomy should include:
   a. Hyperinflation of the lungs
   b. Instilling normal saline into the tube
   c. Suctioning for more than 15 seconds
   d. Tracheostomy care once daily
3. Normal circulation can be maintained in the neurologic patient by:
   a. High-dose heparin therapy
   b. Encouraging ambulation
   c. Active and passive exercises
   d. Dangling limbs in the dependent position
4. Orthostatic hypotension can be minimized by:
   a. Gradually raising the head of the bed
   b. Administering antihypotensive drugs
   c. Slowly adjusting the patient's position
   d. Encouraging the use of a tilt table
5. To prevent musculoskeletal complications in the patient with impaired mobility, you should:
   a. Keep splints on at all times
   b. Keep the patient sitting as long as possible
   c. Maintain proper body alignment
   d. Carry out active and passive exercises
6. Fluid restriction may be necessary for the neurologic patient if:
   a. Diabetes insipidus is suspected
   b. Specific gravity of the urine is below 1.005
   c. Cerebral edema is present
   d. The patient's mobility is decreased

7. In order to promote adequate dietary intake, you should:
   a. Assess the patient's food preferences
   b. Offer large meals
   c. Sit with the patient while he eats
   d. Encourage liquid food in patients with dysphagia
8. When giving an intermittent tube feeding, you should:
   a. Elevate the head of the bed 30 degrees
   b. Check the position of the tube
   c. Withhold feeding if more than 30 ml are aspirated from the patient's stomach
   d. Maintain patient in an upright position for an hour after feeding
9. Managing a patient with altered urinary elimination should include:
   a. Forcing fluids, if possible
   b. Insertion of an internal catheter
   c. Offering the bed pan or urinal frequently
   d. Use of adult diapers
10. For a patient with expressive aphasia, which of the following would you do?
    a. Speak clearly, in short phrases
    b. Use an alphabet board
    c. Speak loudly
    d. Correct all the patient's errors

ANSWERS
1. a, d, e.
2. a, b.
3. b, c.
4. a, c.
5. c, d.
6. c.
7. a, c.
8. b, d.
9. a, c.
10. a, b.

CHAPTER 6

Seizures

OBJECTIVES

After completing this chapter, you will be able to:

1. Discuss the etiology of seizure disorders
2. Classify seizure disorders according to their clinical and electroencephalographic manifestations
3. Describe the usual diagnostic studies performed to determine the type and cause of a seizure disorder
4. Identify the factors that may precipitate a seizure
5. Name the indications and side effects of major anticonvulsant medications
6. List safety precautions to be employed in caring for an epileptic patient
7. Discuss the educational needs of the patient with epilepsy
8. Identify the causes of status epilepticus.

A. Introduction

A *seizure* is the result of the firing of numerous brain cells. It consists of involuntary movements of the body, changes in mental functioning, or a combination of both. A seizure is a symptom of a more complex problem. *Epilepsy* exists when seizures begin to recur without identifiable etiology. Epilepsy is therefore a chronic syndrome. Often the terms epilepsy, seizures, and seizure disorders are used interchangeably.

An estimated 1 million to 4 million Americans suffer from epilepsy. This condition is more common in children and adults over 50, but can occur at any age and in all races and both sexes. Approximately 70 percent of epileptic patients have their first seizure before the age of 20. As epileptics grow older, the type of seizure varies with age.

B. Etiology

It is still not known whether epilepsy is an inherited disorder, but it has been theorized that some individuals have a lower neuronal threshold, which predisposes them to seizures.

1. Idiopathic epilepsy

This type of epilepsy has an undeterminable cause, because the patient has no identifiable cerebellar lesion or metabolic disorder. It was once called "true epilepsy."

2. Acquired epilepsy

This type of epilepsy is caused by a pathologic condition. As many as 50 disorders are known to cause seizures. These disorders can be cerebral, biochemical, or post-traumatic.

a. Cerebral disorders. Cerebral disorders account for a large number of conditions that can cause seizures. These include cerebral damage before or during birth; trauma to the head; intracranial hemorrhages; infectious disorders such as meningitis, abscesses, or high fever; cerebrovascular accidents and cerebral circulatory problems; cerebral edema; degenerative disorders; space-occupying lesions; cerebral anoxia; and congenital malformations.

b. Biochemical disorders. A large variety of disorders that affect the body's biochemical makeup can cause seizures. These include toxic levels of alcohol, drugs, lead, etc.; electrolyte imbalances; disorders of glucose metabolism; vitamin deficiency; and eclampsia.

c. Post-traumatic epilepsy. Seizures may develop several months or even years after cerebral trauma, most commonly between 6 months and 2 years.

d. Precipitating factors. Although the stimuli that trigger a seizure can vary from person to person, there is usually one specific factor for a particular individual. Fever, exhaustion, drugs, alcohol, photosensitivity, hyperventilation, menses, and trauma can precipitate a seizure. Increases in emotional stress can also trigger seizure activity in a susceptible individual.

e. Age. Between birth and the age of 6 months, the most common causes of seizures are birth injuries, infections, and congenital defects. Up to the age of 20, idiopathic seizures are most often seen. In young adulthood, 20 to 30 years of age, structural damage, perhaps the result of trauma or tumor, has been the major cause of seizures. Cerebrovascular diseases and tumors account for seizures in the over-50 age group.

C. Classification of seizures

The most practical system used to classify seizures is the International Classification of Epileptic Seizures (Gastaut, 1970). This system is based on the clinical and electroencephalographic nature of seizures, dividing them into two major types: partial and generalized. Both types are then subdivided further.

1. Partial seizures

This type of seizure is the result of a lesion on the brain. The patient usually experiences an aura, which varies according to the focus of the brain from where the seizure originates. An aura can be a hallucination (visual, auditory, olfactory, or vertiginous), an illusion (distortion of objects or people), a dyscognitive state (feeling of familiarity or unfamiliarity), or an affective experience (fear or anxiety).

Partial seizures can be simple or complex. If the hyperactivity originates at one focus but spreads throughout the brain, it is then termed a *secondary generalized seizure*.

a. Simple partial seizures. This type of seizure depends on the focus of the brain where it originates. If the focus is in the area of the motor strip, the result is a *focal motor seizure*. Symptoms include focal twitching, which may or may not spread to other muscles. Should the seizure spread to other muscles, it is then called "jacksonian march," after the neurologist who first described the attack.

Partial seizures that involve the sensory areas of the brain are termed *focal sensory seizures*. In these, the seizure is felt as tingling or numbness, or there may be visual, auditory, vertiginous, or olfactory sensations, depending on the area of the brain involved. Neither focal motor nor focal sensory seizures involve loss of consciousness.

A secondary generalized partial seizure resembles a generalized major motor seizure (grand mal) with associated coma afterward. However, after the seizure, transient weakness or paralysis may occur (Todd's paralysis), in contrast to a generalized major motor seizure.

b. Complex partial seizures. This type of seizure was once termed temporal lobe seizure, after the part of the brain where such attacks begin. The attack often begins with an aura. The seizure may consist of bizarre motor, sensory, behavioral, or autonomic symptoms. Any interference with the patient's behavior during the seizure may result in aggressive or violent responses. The seizure may last anywhere from a few minutes to several hours, and end abruptly with the patient being amnesic, confused, and drowsy. This type of seizure can progress to a secondary generalized, major motor seizure.

2. Generalized seizures

Both hemispheres of the brain are activated in this type of seizure. The seizure activity is bilateral and symmetrical. During the seizure the patient loses consciousness.

a. Tonic-clonic seizures (grand mal). The grand mal seizure begins with loss of consciousness (usually not preceded by an aura), followed by the tonic phase. The patient falls with arms and legs extended, the jaw snaps shut, the eyes roll back, and the pupils dilate; the patient is apneic and incontinent of urine and feces. The tonic phase lasts less than 1 minute. The clonic phase then begins with violent muscular contractions, hyperventilation, excessive salivation, sweating, and rapid pulse. The entire seizure can last 2 to 5 minutes. Afterward, the patient may fall into a deep sleep and awake confused, with no memory of the event. Injuries may be sustained from the fall. When the patient experiences a second grand mal seizure without fully regaining consciousness from the first, the condition is called *status epilepticus*. Emergency medical treatment is essential to prevent permanent brain damage. Table 6-1 summarizes nursing responsibilities during and immediately after a grand mal seizure.

b. Absence seizures (petit mal). These seizures usually occur in children between the ages of 5 and 12 years and

---

TABLE 6-1

NURSING RESPONSIBILITY DURING
A TONIC-CLONIC (GRAND MAL) SEIZURE

Stay with the patient
Remain calm
Help patient lie down
If patient is lying on floor, don't move him unless in danger
Remove dangerous objects from area
Place padded tongue blade or cloth between unclenched teeth, but don't force it
Loosen constrictive clothing
Do not restrain movements
Elevate patient's head on pillow or your lap
Turn patient on side or turn head
Insert oral airway if possible
Allow secretions to drain, or suction airway
Reorient patient when awake
Make pertinent observations

often stop during the teen-age years. The attacks occur suddenly, with a momentary loss of consciousness that lasts about 5 to 10 seconds. During the attack the child appears to be daydreaming, his eyes become vacant, and he is unresponsive if spoken to. The patient is usually unaware of the seizures, which can occur anywhere from several times to hundreds of times daily.

c. Myoclonic seizures. Myoclonic seizures are characterized by brief, rapid, bilateral jerking of the extremities, without loss of consciousness.

d. Atonic seizures. This type of seizure occurs without an aura. It is characterized by a loss of muscle tone without loss of consciousness. During the seizure the patient falls to the ground. The seizure lasts only a second.

3. Status epilepticus

When a patient has two or more seizures in succession, the condition is called status epilepticus. It is a major medical emergency if tonic-clonic seizures are involved, because cerebral anoxia may result from impaired respiration and cause brain damage or death. The chances of aspiration also increase.

The major cause of status epilepticus is the abrupt cessation of anticonvulsant medications. Fever, meningitis, brain abscess, trauma, certain medications, and drug overdose are also precipitating factors. Treatment is directed toward maintaining respirations, preventing complications and breaking the status with the use of medications such as diazepam (Valium).

D. Diagnosis

In addition to an accurate seizure diagnosis, the underlying cause and precipitating factors must be determined. The most important aspect of an accurate diagnosis is obtaining a complete description of the seizure from the patient himself as well as from witnesses of the attack. Refer to Chapter 2 for details on obtaining a seizure history. Also important is a complete physical and neurologic exam. The most important diagnostic procedure is the electroencephalogram (EEG), which can identify electrical patterns of the brain that correlate with the particular type of seizure. The EEG is also used to localize a seizure-producing lesion or focus if one exists. Other studies may be utilized to determine whether a systemic or central nervous system disorder is the cause of the seizure activity: CT scans, skull X-rays, lumbar puncture, cerebral arteriogram, blood studies to determine the possible presence of metabolic problems or infection, and electrocardiogram.

E. Nursing assessment

Most patients with a seizure disorder are admitted to the hospital either because they have just experienced their first seizure or because their seizures cannot be controlled. One of your goals in these situations is to make pertinent observations as to what occurred during the seizure so that an accurate diagnosis can be made.

1. Seizure history

The information needed for a complete seizure history is found in Chapter 2. If the patient cannot remember all details of the seizure, question others present who may have witnessed it. It is important to determine what may have precipitated the attack, so question the patient as to whether he is taking any anticonvulsants, what the dosage is, whether he's been taking them regularly, and whether he has started to take any other types of medications. Ask also whether the patient has noticed any change in his physical health or if his life has recently become more stressful. Once a complete history has been obtained, you should identify the patient's problems and goals for care.

Carefully record observations of the attack, particularly if the type of seizure has yet to be determined. The following questions should serve as a guide in describing the seizure:
- What was the patient doing before the attack?
- During the attack, was he alert or unresponsive?
- In what part of the body did the seizure begin?
- Were the movements bilateral or unilateral?

- What were the movements like?
- Was there any chewing, lipsmacking, or fluttering of eyelids?
- Did the patient cry out?
- Did the head or eyes turn to one side?
- What were the pupillary reactions?
- Was there cyanosis, frothing at the mouth, tongue biting, or incontinence?
- What did the patient do after the seizure?
- Did he sleep or offer any complaints?
- Was there paralysis?
- What does the patient remember about his seizure?

2. Emotional support

Understandably, the patient who has just experienced his first seizure is usually frightened by what has happened, and by the possibility that it may happen again. The patient who has experienced a seizure after having had his attacks under control for a long period of time will be equally upset. Spend time with the patient, encouraging him to ask questions and to vent his fears so that a relationship of trust can be established. To help alleviate his fears, explain the diagnostic procedures and tests that he'll undergo, and offer reassurance as needed.

3. Seizure precautions

When a patient is subject to seizures, safety becomes a primary concern. Table 6-2 lists general seizure precautions.

TABLE 6-2

SAFETY PRECAUTIONS FOR SEIZURE PATIENTS

Keep bed in low position
Keep side rails up; pad them if necessary
Keep padded tongue blade, oral airway, and suction equipment nearby
Take temperatures by the rectal or axillary route if seizures are poorly controlled
Have the patient take showers instead of baths
Allow no unsupervised smoking

4. Assessing treatment outcomes

If an identifiable cause of seizures is found, your nursing care will obviously depend on its treatment. Nevertheless, you should continue to observe for seizure activity and maintain seizure precautions throughout the patient's hospitalization.

If no cause for the seizures can be determined, anticonvulsant drug therapy will most likely be instituted (such therapy may even be given prophylactically in those patients whose seizure cause has been found). Administer the drugs as ordered and check the patient continually for any symptoms of drug toxicity. Table 6-3 lists the most commonly used anticonvulsant drugs and pertinent information for assessment.

Common signs of anticonvulsant drug toxicity include diplopia, ataxia, drowsiness, and mental dullness. Periodically perform a neurologic assessment, and include the following points in your exam: testing extraocular movements for nystagmus; determining the presence of diplopia; evaluating coordination by finger-to-nose movement, tandem walking, and Romberg's test; and assessing mental acuity. If signs of toxicity appear, the dosage will be lowered or another drug will be prescribed.

5. Patient education

Patient teaching is an important adjunct to assessment. It should begin as soon as the patient is admitted to the hospital. Tailor your teaching plan to the patient's needs and lifestyle, taking into account his social, psychological, vocational, and physical needs. Include the patient's family in your discussions, since they will need help in adjusting to his condition and must know what to do if a seizure occurs.

Begin by making sure that the patient understands his specific seizure disorder, the anticonvulsant drugs he must take, their dosage, time of administration, and possible side effects. Explain the necessity of compliance with the regimen, and that stopping his medications abruptly can trigger status epilepticus.

TABLE 6-3

MAJOR ANTICONVULSANT DRUGS

Medication and adult dosage	Indication	Therapeutic serum level	Side effects
Phenobarbital 60-200 mg/day	All types of seizures	10-30 µg/ml	Drowsiness, vertigo, rash, GI symptoms
Primidone (Mysoline) 250-500 mg/day	All partial seizures, generalized tonic-clonic	5-12 µg/ml	Drowsiness, ataxia, nystagmus, GI symptoms, anemia, rash
Phenytoin (Dilantin) 300-600 mg/day	All partial seizures, generalized tonic-clonic; not used with absence seizures	10-25 µg/ml	Nystagmus, ataxia, confusion, diplopia, drowsiness, GI symptoms, rash, gingival hyperplasia, blood dyscrasias
Carbamazepine (Tegretol) 600-1,800 mg/day	All partial seizures, generalized tonic-clonic, absence seizures	5-12 µg/ml	Dizziness, drowsiness, nausea and vomiting, blood dyscrasias, rash
Clonazepam (Clonopin) 2-20 mg/day	Akinetic, myoclonic, absence seizures	13-72 ng/ml*	Drowsiness, ataxia, behavior problems, blood dyscrasias, rash
Diazepam (Valium) 5-10 mg IV	Drug of choice for status epilepticus		Drowsiness, ataxia
Ethosuximide (Zarontin) 750-1,500 mg/day	Absence seizures	40-100 µg/ml	Drowsiness, dizziness, nausea and vomiting, blood dyscrasias
Trimethadione (Tridione) 900-2,100 mg/day	Absence seizures	600-800 µg/ml	Drowsiness, dizziness, gastric distress, blurred vision, diplopia, blood dyscrasias
Valproic acid (Depakene) 800-2,000 mg/day	Absence seizures	50-100 µg/ml	Drowsiness, anorexia, nausea and vomiting, rash, ataxia, blood dyscrasias

*One nanogram = 1/1,000,000 milligram.

Discuss factors that trigger seizures, and how best the patient can avoid them. In particular, tell the patient to avoid fatigue, constipation, and stress, to limit fluids and caffeine, and to avoid alcohol completely.

Women should know that menses often trigger seizure activity. If a patient is of childbearing age and wants to have a baby, advise her to discuss this with her physician, since anticonvulsant drugs can affect the fetus.

Stress the importance of physical activity, which tends to inhibit rather than increase seizures. Tell the patient that he can take part in most activities, but should avoid those in which he could be harmed if a seizure occurred.

Finally, the patient should obtain a Medic Alert bracelet or necklace and carry a card that identifies his condition, physician, hospital, medications and dosage, and any allergies he may have.

QUIZ

1. The type of epilepsy that appears to have no determined cause is _____ epilepsy.

2. List the three types of disorders that can cause acquired epilepsy:

3. Which of the following is *not* considered a precipitating factor in seizures?
   a. Menses
   b. Allergies
   c. Stress
   d. Alcohol
   e. Photosensitivity

Match the seizure classification with the symptoms each exhibits.

4. Focal motor seizure ____
5. Focal sensory seizure ____
6. Secondary generalized partial seizure ____
7. Complex partial seizure ____
8. Tonic-clonic seizure ____
9. Absence seizure ____
10. Myoclonic seizure ____
11. Atonic seizure ____

a. Momentary loss of consciousness of 5 to 10 seconds
b. Loss of muscle tone without loss of consciousness
c. Abnormal sensations
d. Abnormal movements begin in a specific area and spread throughout the body
e. Bizarre motor or sensory behavior or autonomic symptoms
f. Loss of consciousness followed by tonic and clonic phases
g. Brief, rapid bilateral jerking of extremities without loss of consciousness
h. Focal twitching in a body part

12. Common toxic effects of anticonvulsant therapy include _____, _____, _____, and _____.

13. The drug of choice for status epilepticus is _____.

14. List three areas you should include in teaching epileptic patients:

15. Status epilepticus is most commonly triggered by _____ and _____.

ANSWERS
1. Idiopathic.
2. Cerebral disorders, biochemical disorders, trauma.
3. b.
4. h.
5. c.
6. d.
7. e.
8. f.
9. a.
10. g.
11. b.
12. Diplopia; ataxia; drowsiness; mental dullness.
13. Valium.
14. Information regarding the patient's specific seizure disorder, anticonvulsant drug regimen, precipitating factors, diet, pregnancy, activity, Medic Alert identification.
15. Stopping anticonvulsant medications; fever.

CHAPTER

Cerebrovascular Diseases

OBJECTIVES

After completing this chapter, you will be able to:

1. Identify the factors that predispose a person to stroke
2. Discuss the pathophysiology and classification of strokes
3. Correlate the signs and symptoms of stroke with the specific occluded vessel
4. Identify the common deficits in left- and right-sided hemiplegia
5. Discuss the pathophysiology and complications of cerebral aneurysms and arteriovenous malformations
6. Describe subarachnoid precautions
7. Describe nursing assessment and management principles for these disorders.

A. Cerebrovascular accident (stroke)

Cerebrovascular accident, or stroke, is the third leading cause of death in the United States, and affects more than 1 million Americans each year. It occurs more frequently in the elderly over age 65, in men, and in blacks. There is also a tendency for stroke to run in certain families.

1. Definition of cerebrovascular accident

A cerebrovascular accident is the name for a variety of neurologic deficits that occur suddenly as a result of inadequate blood supply to an area of the brain. The symptoms of a stroke can range from a mild tingling or weakness of an extremity to complete loss of consciousness, hemiplegia, and/or aphasia. It is important to recognize that a stroke is a syndrome, since the cause may vary; it is not a disease entity in itself.

2. Predisposing factors

The main factor known to put individuals at risk of stroke is hypertension. Other predisposing conditions include atherosclerotic changes, diabetes mellitus, obesity, high levels of serum cholesterol, lipoproteins, and triglycerides, cigarette smoking, use of oral contraceptives, stress, heart disease, collagen disease, and a sedentary lifestyle.

3. Pathophysiology of stroke

The brain has protective mechanisms for assuring a continuous supply of blood and nutrients. Its arteries are interconnected by the circle of Willis (see Figure 1-5) so that if one vessel becomes occluded, the rest will take over. However, as many as half the population are thought to have an anomaly of the circle of Willis, so this mechanism is not always effective. There are also homeostatic mechanisms within the brain that maintain cerebral blood flow at approximately 800 ml/minute, assuring a constant supply of glucose and oxygen. These mechanisms, however, can fail if subjected to a large amount of stress.

If a thrombus or embolus cuts off the blood supply to an area of the brain, infarction of brain tissue can result. The loss of blood to a specific area for more than 3 minutes can cause permanent brain damage, because neurons cannot regenerate. Further damage to the area can result from cerebral edema, which compresses surrounding capillaries.

B. Classification of strokes
1. Thrombotic stroke

Most strokes are caused by the formation of a thrombus from atherosclerotic plaque, which has narrowed the vessel wall. In a stroke, the thrombus may at first occlude the lumen only partially, but may advance to complete occlusion in a matter of hours or days. Thrombotic strokes are further classified as transient ischemic attacks, stroke-in-evolution, or completed stroke.

a. Transient ischemic attacks (TIA). A transient ischemic attack produces a focal neurologic deficit that can last anywhere from a few minutes to hours, then disappears. Such attacks are often a prelude to a stroke, and can be experienced any number of times. The symptoms of a TIA depend on the specific arteries involved. Table 7-1 outlines

TABLE 7-1

SYMPTOMS OF TRANSIENT ISCHEMIC ATTACKS

Carotid artery
  Paresis (contralateral monoparesis to hemiplegia)
  Sensory deficits (contralateral)
  Vision loss or deficit
  Dysphasia
  Dysarthria
  Confusion
Vertebrobasilar system
  Vertigo
  Visual deficits
  Paresthesia
  Paresis
  Dysarthria
  Ataxia
  Headache
  Nausea/vomiting

the symptoms that can occur with lesions of the carotid artery and vertebrobasilar system, the most common sites of atherosclerosis in the extracranial arteries.

The diagnosis of TIA begins with a patient history that details when the initial attack occurred, its description, how often it occurs, and when it was experienced last. After a complete physical, the patient undergoes diagnostic testing that includes tomography of the head and neck, cerebral angiography, and cerebral blood flow studies. The testing determines whether the lesion is in an extracranial vessel, such as the internal carotid, or in an intracranial artery, such as the middle cerebral artery, the most common site of atherosclerosis of the intracranial arteries. Extensive testing helps determine whether surgery is necessary. Carotid endarterectomy and superior temporal artery-middle cerebral artery anastomosis are two surgical procedures currently utilized in the treatment of TIA to improve blood circulation to the brain.

b. Stroke-in-evolution. Occasionally the symptoms of stroke evolve gradually over hours or days. The symptoms may improve temporarily, only to worsen a short time later. This condition is termed *stroke-in-evolution*, and is an acute emergency usually treated with large doses of heparin. It may be necessary to perform emergency angiography and, possibly, surgery.

c. Completed stroke. This term describes the stable, usually permanent symptoms of stroke.

2. Embolic stroke

An embolic stroke most often occurs from the breaking apart of a coronary thrombus, whose fragments are carried to the brain. This type of stroke may be precipitated by mitral stenosis, atrial flutter, fibrillation, myocardial infarction, and bacterial endocarditis. Less common causes of embolic stroke are fat or tumor-cell emboli, and emboli that result from cardiac or vascular surgery.

An embolic stroke occurs rapidly—sometimes within seconds—and gives no prior warning. The embolus can stay lodged at one site or break up and obstruct smaller vessels. The resultant symptoms will depend on the artery or arteries involved.

3. Hemorrhagic stroke

The most common causes of hemorrhagic stroke include hypertensive intracranial hemorrhage, ruptured cerebral aneurysm, ruptured arteriovenous malformation, trauma, and hemorrhagic diseases (e.g., liver disease, leukemia, hemophilia). Like embolic stroke, hemorrhagic stroke occurs rapidly, with possible symptoms of headache, vomiting, nuchal rigidity, and focal signs depending on the area of brain involvement. Most hemorrhagic strokes occur in the area of the basal ganglia and subcortical white matter. Other areas affected include the thalamus, cerebellum, and pons.

C. Prognosis in stroke

Massive thrombotic stroke can cause severe cerebral edema that could result in brain stem herniation and death. In less severe strokes, cerebral edema may last only a few days, with recovery taking place in a matter of hours or weeks. Recovery depends on how much of the brain was affected, what area was involved, and whether any pathologic changes have remained.

The prognosis for embolic stroke is similar to that of thrombotic stroke. If the embolus breaks up, the signs and symptoms of stroke may disappear, but unless the underlying disease is treated, more strokes may occur.

In a major hemorrhagic stroke, coma and death may result. Smaller hemorrhages may lead to clot formation producing the symptoms of a stroke until the clot is slowly absorbed.

D. Symptoms of stroke

The signs and symptoms of stroke depend on the area and extent of damage.

1. Middle cerebral artery occlusion

This is the most common cerebral vessel to become occluded. If the main stem of this vessel is blocked, infarction of the cerebral hemisphere occurs. Symptoms seen with this syndrome include contralateral hemiplegia and anesthesia, aphasia with dominant side involvement, homonymous hemianopsia, alterations in level of consciousness, and lack of recognition of the paralyzed side.

2. Anterior cerebral artery occlusion

The anterior cerebral artery is rarely occluded, but when occlusion occurs, symptoms include paralysis and sensory loss in the contralateral foot and leg, paresis of the contralateral arm, gait problems, urinary incontinence, abulia (inability to perform voluntary acts or make decisions), distractability, lack of interest in surroundings, amnesia, and contralateral grasp and sucking reflexes.

3. Posterior cerebral artery occlusion

This occurs in roughly 3 percent of cerebral occlusions. Symptoms of this syndrome vary considerably, and can include contralateral sensory loss, contralateral homonymous hemianopsia, memory loss, mild contralateral hemiparesis, color blindness, lack of depth perception, intentional tremors, and ipsilateral third-nerve palsy with contralateral hemiplegia or ataxia.

4. Internal carotid artery occlusion

The patient with occlusion of an internal carotid artery may exhibit few symptoms if adequate anastomotic circulation exists. If symptoms do arise, they generally consist of transient blindness in the ipsilateral eye, contralateral weakness and paresthesia in the arm, face, and leg, contralateral hemiplegia with sensory loss, and dysphasia.

5. Posterior inferior cerebellar artery occlusion

Occlusion of this artery can cause infarction of the lateral portion of the medulla. Symptoms of this syndrome include ipsilateral loss of pain and temperature sensation in the face, dysphagia, dysarthria, contralateral loss of pain and temperature sensation in the trunk and limbs, ataxia, vertigo, horizontal nystagmus, and ipsilateral Horner's syndrome (miosis, ptosis, decreased sweating).

6. Anterior inferior cerebellar artery occlusion

Occlusion of this artery results in pontine involvement. Symptoms include ipsilateral deafness and tinnitus, vertigo, nausea, vomiting, nystagmus, ataxia, ipsilateral Horner's syndrome, and contralateral pain and temperature loss.

E. Deficits in left- and right-sided hemiplegia

The type of disabilities a patient will be left with after a stroke depends, in part, on whether he is right- or left-handed, and on which side of the brain the stroke occurred. Right-handed individuals have their dominant cerebral hemisphere on the left, while left-handed individuals have their dominant cerebral hemisphere on the right. In 60 percent of left-handed individuals, however, the speech center is located in the left hemisphere. Table 7-2 outlines specific functional deficits as they relate to the two hemispheres of the brain.

F. Diagnosis of stroke

A thorough history and physical exam are necessary for accurate diagnosis of the stroke syndrome. It's important to identify the cause of the stroke in order to plan effective treatment. Diagnostic studies often used to determine the underlying cause include lumbar puncture, computed

TABLE 7-2

FUNCTIONAL DEFICITS IN RIGHT AND LEFT HEMIPLEGIA

Right hemiplegia	*Left hemiplegia*
Expressive and/or receptive aphasia	Perceptive impairment
Frustration and depression	Neglect of affected side
Difficulty distinguishing left from right	Lack of inhibitions, inappropriate behavior
Decreased intellectual performance	Inability to recognize faces
Right homonymous hemianopsia	Left homonymous hemianopsia
	Poor judgment

tomography (CT scan), cerebral angiography, brain scan, and electroencephalogram.

G. Medical management of stroke

Medical management of the acute phase of a cerebrovascular accident — usually the first 24 to 48 hours — consists of support and maintenance of all vital body functions. Efforts are focused on maintaining an airway, fluid and electrolyte balance, cerebral perfusion, and temperature. Dexamethasone sodium phosphate (Decadron phosphate) and/or mannitol may be given to decrease cerebral edema.

Anticoagulants are not effective in a completed stroke but may be given for a stroke-in-evolution and to prevent further embolic strokes.

Once the cause of the stroke is determined, attempts are made to control or eliminate the cause. Surgery, such as carotid endarterectomy or bypass, may be performed if the occlusion is incomplete. Rehabilitation is begun on admission, and the patient is encouraged to become more actively involved in his care as his condition improves.

H. Nursing assessment of the stroke patient

1. Acute phase

During the first 24 to 48 hours following a stroke, your assessment of the patient is important. Assess respiratory function through frequent auscultation and evaluation of arterial blood gases.

Frequent observation of neurologic status includes assessing level of consciousness and evaluating pupillary signs, extraocular movement, cranial nerve, motor, and sensory functions, and reflexes.

Monitor vital signs for any abnormalities that could indicate respiratory or cardiac changes.

Evaluate fluid and electrolyte balance by assessing intake and output. Measure output every 1 to 2 hours. Check urine specific gravity. Monitor blood electrolytes for abnormalities.

Assess for any seizure activity and be sure to implement seizure precautions.

2. Postacute phase

After the acute phase of stroke, monitor vital and neurologic signs routinely. Continue to assess airway patency and respiratory function, and assess skin integrity and musculoskeletal status. Evaluate bowel and bladder elimination for any alterations that require intervention. Assess swallowing ability and monitor food and fluid intake. Evaluate the presence and extent of communication and visual, perceptual, and intellectual deficits.

Observe for possible complications such as paralytic ileus (check bowel sounds), infection (fever), pulmonary embolus (chest pain and respiratory alteration), and myocardial infarction (chest pain, arm pain, breathing difficulties, etc.).

Be sure to review all diagnostic studies for abnormalities.

I. Nursing management of the stroke patient

During the acute phase, your immediate goal is to maintain the patient's vital functions. Your care must include measures to maintain a patent airway, fluid and electrolyte balance, cerebral blood flow, and safety. Begin general nursing measures to prevent complications of immobility. If the patient is unconscious, include the appropriate nursing care.

During the postacute phase, direct your care toward preventing complications and preparing for rehabilitation. Continue to maintain adequate respiratory function. Skin care and general hygiene are important. Prevent musculoskeletal complications, promote nutrition and hydration, maintain proper elimination, and provide for patient safety. The presence of specific deficits requires special management techniques.

Refer to Chapter 5 for specific information on meeting the neurologic patient's needs.

J. Assessment for discharge planning

This process occurs throughout the stroke patient's hospitalization. The entire health team must be involved in planning. Included in the plan should be the types of activities the patient can participate in. Discourage the family from introducing unfamiliar activities, hobbies, and games that may cause him frustration.

Discuss with the family and patient the risk factors for stroke, as well as prodromal symptoms such as dizziness, headaches, and numbness. Encourage them to obtain treatment quickly to prevent completion of another stroke. Bring up the topic of sexual activity to both patient and spouse, first with each separately and then together. They may each have unasked questions and unexpressed concerns. Other areas include equipment needed at home and help available through community services. Going home on a pass can give the patient and family a trial run so that problems can be identified and dealt with.

If the patient is to be discharged to a nursing home or rehabilitation center, a plan of care should be sent to that facility. Discharge can be both a happy and a frightening experience for the patient and family. Your support, encouragement, and teaching can help them make a smooth transition.

K. Cerebral aneurysms

A cerebral aneurysm is a saclike dilation of the arterial vessel that develops from a weakness in the internal and middle layers of the wall. The more common type, berry aneurysms, are so called because, like berries, they have a stem and a neck. Saccular aneurysms balloon from the vessel and have no neck.

Most aneurysms are small, approximately 1 cm in diameter, although some are capable of dilating as much as 5 cm. They usually develop in the anterior portion of the circle of Willis, and are especially common at the juncture of the posterior communicating artery and internal carotid artery. Not all aneurysms are harmful; in many patients they remain silent for life.

1. Etiology of aneurysms

Although the exact cause of aneurysms is not known, several theories have been proposed. Among them are congenital defects of the cerebral arteries, arteriosclerosis, hypertension, and trauma to the head.

2. Signs and symptoms of aneurysms

Cerebral aneurysms occur most often in individuals aged 35 to 60. Symptoms before rupture, experienced by about half of all patients, include headache, lethargy, neck pain, and sometimes dysfunction of the optic, oculomotor, or trigeminal nerve. Specific symptoms depend on the location and size of the aneurysm.

After rupture or bleeding, symptoms include violent, "explosive" headache, decreased consciousness, deficits of the cranial nerves, muscular and visual disturbances, vomiting, nuchal rigidity, vertigo, irritability, and fever. The symptoms and their severity depend on the extent and location of the bleed. Rupture of an aneurysm is obviously a life-threatening situation.

3. Diagnosis of aneurysms

After a preliminary physical exam, diagnosis of a cerebral aneurysm is made with the help of a number of diagnostic studies, including cerebral arteriogram (the most valuable indicator), lumbar puncture, CT scan, and, if necessary, an electroencephalogram and brain scan.

4. Progression and complications

The patient is at great risk of death if, during rupture of a cerebral aneurysm, he loses more than 30 ml of blood before a clot forms. If he survives the initial bleed, the patient is still in danger of two threatening complications: rebleeding and vasospasms.

a. Rebleeding. Rebleeding occurs when the clot at the aneurysm site dissolves before the tissue is fully healed. Forty percent of patients will experience a rebleed after an aneurysm rupture, most commonly from the third to the 11th day after the initial bleed.

b. Vasospasms. A cerebral vasospasm is a focal constriction of the arteries of the circle of Willis or its main branches. The narrowing occurs most often in the vessel adjacent to the ruptured aneurysm, and can cause ischemia of the cerebral tissue supplied by the vessel. Ischemia can lead to infarction or death. Vasospasms can occur even after successful surgery.

Symptoms of vasospasm depend on the area involved but often include a decreased level of consciousness, hemiparesis, and visual disturbances. Observation for seizure activity is also necessary.

L. Medical management of the patient with cerebral aneurysm

Because surgery for cerebral aneurysm often is not successful immediately after the bleed, it is delayed for 5 days to several weeks. Conservative management is utilized until the patient's condition stabilizes. The goals of therapy are to prevent complications and improve or maintain the patient's neurologic status. Drug therapy during this time may include the following:
- Antihypertensives – used if hypertension exists
- Anti-inflammatory agent – dexamethasone to decrease cerebral edema
- Antifibrolytic – aminocaproic acid (Amicar) to prevent rebleeding by preventing destruction of the clot
- Antivasospasm agent – reserpine (Serpasil), kanamycin (Kantrex), or isoproterenol (Isuprel) and aminophylline in combination
- Sedatives – to prevent excitement and increase in blood pressure.

M. Nursing assessment and management of aneurysm patients

1. Neurologic assessment

The baseline assessment should evaluate the patient's level of consciousness, pupillary signs, and motor, sensory, and cranial nerve function, and should determine the presence of headache, nuchal rigidity, blurred vision, or aphasia. Make frequent checks of the patient's neurologic and vital signs, particularly during the acute stage after rupture.

2. Subarachnoid precautions

It is essential for the patient to rest in a quiet environment with lights dim, so that he remains calm and his blood pressure stays low. The head of the bed should be elevated at least 30 degrees, with an alternating-pressure or egg-crate mattress provided.

All basic daily care, including feeding and bathing, should be performed for the patient, to prevent exertion that would raise his blood pressure or promote straining. He should be cautioned not to turn himself or pull himself up in bed, as this would initiate Valsalva's maneuver, increasing intracranial pressure. Instead, turn him from side to side every 2 hours to prevent skin breakdown and respiratory problems. The patient should also be warned against coughing, sneezing, blowing his nose, or straining.

Apply antiembolic stockings to prevent thrombophlebitis, and give medication for headache as needed to prevent restlessness. Stool softeners and mild laxatives may be prescribed to avoid constipation.

External stimuli, such as television, radio, or reading, should not be allowed and visitors should be restricted to only two members of the immediate family at one time.

3. Seizure precautions

Because a cerebral aneurysm patient is in danger of seizures, keep a suction setup, a padded tongue blade, and an oral airway nearby. Maintain other safety precautions.

4. Fluid restrictions

The patient will be restricted to about 1,500 ml of fluid per 24-hour period. To ensure that this amount is not exceeded, maintain an accurate record of intake and output. Make sure the patient and family are made aware of the fluid restriction and the reason for it.

5. Drug therapy

After administering the prescribed medications, assess the patient for his responses and for any signs of drug toxicity. Be familiar with the actions and interactions of other drugs he may be concurrently receiving.

6. Emotional needs

The patient with an aneurysm needs a great deal of emotional support from you. He may be fearful of a rebleed and upcoming surgery in addition to being frustrated by his forced inactivity. Help him remain calm by orienting him to person, place, and time, and by reassuring him about his condition. Watch for any adverse reactions that may result from the restrictions imposed on his activity; in some cases the physician might modify the restrictions. And be supportive of the patient's family.

7. Other nursing measures

Nursing care will depend on the patient's physical condition, which may range from asymptomatic to deeply comatose. Chapter 5 details the specific nursing measures that may be needed.

N. Arteriovenous malformations

An arteriovenous malformation (AVM) is a congenital abnormality of the vasculature of the central nervous system, made up of vessels of early fetal development. Among these thin-walled vessels, there is no distinction among arteries, capillaries, and veins. The arteries feeding an AVM, as well as the veins that drain it, may become engorged and enlarged.

AVMs generally extend from the surface of the brain inward, like a wedge. They are often called shunts, or "steals," because so much oxygenated blood may be shunted through them that cerebral ischemia results. An AVM may compress adjacent cerebral tissue, causing neurologic deficits. AVMs have also caused noncommunicating hydrocephalus and cardiac decompensation. The main danger of an AVM, however, is rupture and hemorrhage through the thin-walled vessels.

1. Incidence

AVMs account for 1 to 6 percent of all subarachnoid hemorrhages. They occur slightly more often in males than in females, and symptoms usually are evident between the ages of 10 and 30.

By age 40, 50 to 75 percent of persons with an AVM have experienced hemorrhage. Once an AVM has bled, whether slightly or severely, there's a 25 percent chance it will rebleed within 4 years.

2. Signs and symptoms

Signs and symptoms of an AVM include those of intracerebral, subarachnoid, or subdural hemorrhage: seizures, headache, motor and sensory losses, aphasia, bruit over the affected area, visual deficits, and mental changes.

3. Diagnosis of AVM

In addition to a complete history, physical, and neurologic exam, the following tests are commonly included in diagnosing AVMs:
- Angiography – the most important test for determining the location and extent of the defect
- Lumbar puncture – evaluates intracranial pressure and reveals the presence of any red cells in CSF; not done if intracranial pressure is already elevated
- Skull films – may show calcification of abnormal vessels
- CT scan – with contrast medium, may differentiate an AVM from a clot or tumor
- Brain scan – injected isotope will be taken up by an AVM.

4. Medical management of patients with AVM

After an AVM has bled, subarachnoid precautions are instituted, since the major complications are rebleeding and vasospasm. Drug therapy is similar to that for an aneurysm rupture. Surgery may involve complete excision, ligation of feeder vessels, or embolization. It usually is postponed for 2 weeks, until the patient's condition is stable.

5. Nursing assessment and management of patients with AVM

Monitor the patient's vital signs and neurologic function. Your goal before surgery is to prevent deterioration in his physical and mental status; after surgery, to help him regain as much independence as possible. Nursing management is similar to that of a patient with a ruptured aneurysm.

QUIZ

1. Which of the following factors predispose a person to stroke?
   a. Hypertension
   b. Headaches
   c. Smoking
   d. Stress
   e. Cancer

2. Loss of blood supply to an area of the brain can result in cerebral _____.

3. List the three types of stroke:

4. Which of the following are symptoms of middle cerebral artery occlusion?
   a. Horner's syndrome
   b. Aphasia
   c. Contralateral hemiplegia
   d. Amnesia
   e. Homonymous hemianopsia

5. Which of the following deficits are usually found with right hemiplegia?
   a. Poor judgment
   b. Aphasia
   c. Depression
   d. Decreased intellectual performance
   e. Perceptual impairment

6. Nursing goals for care of stroke patients during the acute phase include:
   a. Maintaining cerebral blood flow
   b. Monitoring neurologic status
   c. Airway maintenance
   d. Maintaining proper elimination

7. The two major complications of cerebral aneurysms and arteriovenous malformations are _____ and _____.

8. Cerebral aneurysms and AVMs are sometimes treated with drugs. Name three types:

9. Subarachnoid precautions include:

10. Three symptoms of cerebral aneurysm rupture are:

11. The most important tool in diagnosing AVMs is _____.

ANSWERS
1. **a, c, d.**
2. Infarction.
3. Thrombotic, embolic, hemorrhagic.
4. **b, c, e.**
5. **b, c, d.**
6. **a, b, c.**
7. Rebleeding; vasospasm.
8. Antihypertensives; anti-inflammatory agents; antifibrinolytics; antivasospasmotics; sedatives.
9. Turning the radio off; dimming the lights; limiting visitors; preventing exertion; raising head of bed.
10. Violent, "explosive" headache; decreased consciousness; cranial nerve deficits; muscular and visual disturbances; vomiting; nuchal rigidity; vertigo; irritability; fever.
11. Angiography.

CHAPTER

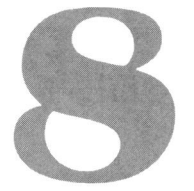

Trauma to the Central Nervous System

OBJECTIVES

After completing this chapter, you will be able to:

1. Discuss the pathophysiology of head injury
2. Describe the types of head injuries
3. Discuss the pathophysiology of spinal cord injury
4. Identify the signs and symptoms of the various types of spinal cord injuries
5. Describe functional loss according to the spinal cord segment involved
6. Discuss nursing assessment and management goals in the care of head- and cord-injured patients
7. Discuss some of the problems involved in rehabilitation of head- and cord-injured patients.

A. Pathophysiology of head injuries

Trauma to the head can be the result of falls, vehicular accidents, industrial accidents, assault, sports accidents, birth injury, electrical accidents, and a variety of other causes.

1. Mechanisms of injury

Head injuries can result from three types of forces: (1) skull deformation, or distortion in the shape of the skull; (2) acceleration-deceleration, where the skull moves faster than the brain mass, resulting in pressure changes; and (3) rotation, where head movement causes rotation and distortion of brain tissue. These forces result in compression, tension, and shearing of brain tissue.

When a moving object strikes the head with sufficient force, a skull fracture results. The fracture may or may not be depressed. The blow can result in contusion of brain tissue at the point of impact, called a *coup* lesion. More often, however, the moving head strikes an immobile structure. Because the skull moves faster than brain tissue, the brain "hits" the skull opposite the site of impact, creating a *contrecoup* lesion.

2. Responses to injury

a. Damage to cerebral tissue. Contusion due to impact may injure nerve cells and fibers and cause small hemorrhages that destroy adjacent tissue. Demyelination of nerve fibers may be followed eventually by regeneration of the myelin sheath.

b. Cerebral edema. Other secondary responses to brain injury include cerebral edema, as increased blood flow forces fluid to move into cerebral tissue. Edema may also occur when some areas of the brain are inadequately perfused and hypercapnia results, leading to local acidosis and vasodilation. An inadequate supply of oxygen and glucose can further increase cerebral edema. Either localized or generalized cerebral edema may increase intracranial pressure to the point of herniation and death.

c. Hemorrhage and hematoma. Shearing forces on brain tissue may cause hemorrhage and hematoma, both leading to increased intracranial pressure. Other responses include ischemia, infarction, and necrosis of brain tissue as well as damage to cranial nerves and other cranial structures.

Any changes in neurologic function will depend on the site, type, and extent of injury.

B. Types of head injuries
1. Skull fractures

Skull fractures can injure the tissues, blood vessels, and nerves of the brain; can tear the dura, causing leakage of cerebrospinal fluid; and, when compound, can open a pathway for intracranial infection.

a. Linear fracture. This is a simple break in bone continuity that does not alter the relationship of the two bone fragments. The patient is observed for cerebral injury.

b. Comminuted fracture. Here the bone is broken into multiple fragments by multiple linear fractures.

c. Depressed fracture. Fragments of bone are indented inward.

d. Compound fracture. Skull fracture involves laceration of the scalp, mucous membranes, paranasal sinuses, eyes, ears, or tympanic membrane. Surgery is needed.

e. Basal skull fractures. These occur at the base of the skull, particularly at the anterior and middle fossae. The fracture can be either linear, comminuted, or depressed. They frequently cause rhinorrhea or otorrhea.

2. Brain injuries

a. Concussion. This is an immediate, transient impairment of neurologic function caused by a blow to the head. There is usually no structural damage, but there may be loss of memory before or after the injury, in addition to lethargy, nausea, and vomiting. Although normal function usually returns, a postconcussion syndrome of headache, dizziness, and inability to concentrate may last for several weeks afterward.

b. Cerebral contusion. Impact causes a structural alteration of the brain's surface that results in bleeding and tissue death, with or without edema. As mentioned, contusions may be coup or contrecoup injuries. They are most common in the frontal and temporal areas. Serious neurologic deficits may result; symptoms depend on the site and extent of damage.

c. Epidural hematoma. An epidural hematoma (extradural hematoma) develops from bleeding into the potential space between the skull and dura mater. This condition typically results from laceration of the middle meningeal artery. With the classic clinical picture, the patient may experience loss of consciousness followed by a lucid period, but his level of consciousness rapidly deteriorates into confusion, coma, and — if untreated — death. However, the lucid interval occurs infrequently; progressive decline in level of consciousness is more common.

d. Subdural hematoma. Arterial or venous bleeding between the dura mater and arachnoid usually produces symptoms within 48 hours if the injury is acute. Common signs and symptoms of *acute* subdural hematoma are headache, drowsiness, agitation, confusion, and dilation and fixation of the ipsilateral pupil. Hemiparesis may occur.

Subacute subdural hematomas produce symptoms similar to those of acute disease, but they develop more slowly — in 2 days to 2 weeks. *Chronic* subdural hematomas are due to minor trauma, and may grow quite large before symptoms are evident. Patients usually present with mental difficulties.

e. Intracerebral hematoma. Intracerebral hematomas are bleeding into the cerebral tissue itself. They usually arise from either deceleration or direct impact injuries, and therefore are most often found in the frontal or temporal lobes. They can also occur deep within the hemispheres, from the shearing effects of rotational movements.

Symptoms include headache, decrease in level of consciousness, contralateral hemiplegia, and ipsilateral pupil dilation.

f. Subarachnoid hemorrhage. Subarachnoid hemorrhage can occur with trauma, although hematoma formation is rare. Signs and symptoms include nuchal rigidity, headache, decreasing level of consciousness, hemiparesis, and ipsilateral dilated pupil.

C. Diagnosis of head injury

The following procedures are commonly used to diagnose the type and extent of trauma in a head-injured patient:

1. Lumbar puncture

This procedure evaluates cerebrospinal fluid pressure and detects the presence of blood. It's contraindicated if there is evidence of increased intracranial pressure.

2. Skull X-ray

This technique identifies skull fractures and metal fragments, although basal skull fractures are not easily diagnosed.

3. CT scan

This is the most important test for the head-injured patient. It's helpful in diagnosing and localizing extracerebral and intracerebral hematomas and contusions.

D. Medical management of the head-injured patient

Medical management of the head-injured patient depends upon the type and extent of the injury and the patient's level of consciousness. Standard medical goals for the severely head-injured patient include:
- Maintenance of airway and ventilation
- Maintenance of blood pressure and temperature
- Prevention of seizures
- Prevention of increased intracranial pressure
- Prevention of infection

- Observation for complications such as inappropriate antidiuretic hormone secretion, diabetes insipidus, and cerebrospinal fluid leaks.

The patient may require surgery immediately or later, after stabilization.

E. Nursing assessment of the head-injured patient

1. Initial assessment

a. Respiratory evaluation. An adequate airway is your primary concern. Assess patency of the airway, adequacy of ventilation, and breathing pattern. As soon as an arterial line has been inserted, measure blood gases.

b. Neurologic assessment. Use the Glasgow coma scale (see Figure 4-1) to assess level of consciousness. A score of 8 or below indicates the need for treatment. Evaluate pupil size and reaction to light. Test the oculocephalic (doll's eyes) response to evaluate brain stem function, and evaluate extraocular movements. Assess cranial nerve, motor, and sensory function and test the patient's deep tendon and Babinski reflexes. Also, evaluate his respiratory pattern. Report any abnormalities or changes from baseline immediately.

c. Vital signs evaluation. Take vital signs frequently. In particular, watch for tachycardia and hypotension, which may indicate hemorrhage outside the nervous system, and for bradycardia and hypertension—late signs of increased intracranial pressure.

d. Other initial measures. Any other non-neurologic traumatic injuries are assessed and treated. Intravenous fluids are begun, and a head wound, if present, is treated. The patient may require immediate surgical treatment.

2. General assessment
- Assess for cerebrospinal fluid leakage from nose or ears
- Basal skull fracture: ecchymosis on mastoid area, periorbital ecchymosis, or conjunctival hemorrhage

- Nuchal rigidity
- Shock, abdominal rigidity, limitation of movement, bruises
- Bowel sounds
- Urinary output and characteristics of urine
- Laboratory studies.

F. Nursing management during the acute phase in the head-injured patient

Nursing care during the acute phase depends on the patient's condition. Patients with severe head trauma and altered consciousness require complex nursing management. Your care in this situation should include maintaining a patent airway and respiratory function, controlling temperature, seizure precautions, skin and eye care and hygiene measures, maintenance of bowel and bladder elimination, and musculoskeletal management. Refer to Chapter 5 for more detailed information. If the head-injured patient undergoes a craniotomy, refer to Chapter 9 for information regarding management.

G. Rehabilitation of the head-injured patient

Care should be taken to maintain any function that is present and prevent complications. The principal goal is restoration of lost function. Neurologic deficits can be similar to those encountered by stroke patients. Refer to Chapter 5 for nursing management of specific deficits. The entire healthcare team works to assess the patient's needs and plan his care. You need to coordinate care and make appropriate referrals. You should also offer support and encouragement to the patient and his family and help them to deal with problems that arise.

H. Pathophysiology of spinal cord injuries

Spinal cord injury is usually the result of vertebral trauma due to direct or indirect impact. Trauma to the vertebrae resulting in fracture or dislocation may or may not cause spinal cord injury. Cord involvement may consist of contusion, stretching of nerve tissue, compression by bone, or complete or partial severance. The areas involved are usually the cervical, lower thoracic, and lumbar regions. The thoracic area is less affected because of the stable protection afforded by the rib cage. Cord injuries are most common in young men between the ages of 15 and 30.

Initially there is paralysis, although no microscopic changes or grossly visible breaks in the cord are seen. Next, small hemorrhages appear in the gray matter and increase until all the gray matter is hemorrhagic and necrotic. Edema occurs in the white matter, with eventual breakdown of myelin and the axon itself. The traumatized segment extends horizontally and vertically. Within 4 hours, the segment is destroyed.

I. Signs and symptoms of spinal cord injury

1. Complete blockage and severance

With complete, abrupt blockage of impulses from higher centers of the brain to the spinal cord cells, *spinal shock* results. Signs and symptoms of spinal shock include:
- Flaccid paralysis below the level of the injury
- Loss of all sensation below the level of the injury
- Loss of spinal reflexes below the level of the injury
- Loss of vasomotor tone, resulting in unstable, lowered blood pressure
- Absence of perspiration below the injury level
- Bladder incontinence and fecal retention.

Spinal shock can last a few days to several months. Recovery is slow. If function below the injury level doesn't return, reflex activity may begin to return. Reflex activity may become so strong that it results in hyperreflexia and spastic paralysis.

Spinal shock does not occur with slow transection of the spinal cord caused by tumors and degenerative neurologic diseases.

2. Partial severance of impulses

Sudden, partial transection can cause spinal shock in those areas involved. Signs and symptoms include:

- Asymmetrical flaccid paralysis below the injury level
- Asymmetrical reflex loss below the injury level
- Some intact sensations below the injury level
- Less vasomotor involvement than in complete blockage or severance
- Less bladder and bowel involvement
- Inability to perspire on one side of the body.

3. Partial cord injury syndromes

a. Anterior cord syndrome. This results from compression of the anterior cord or loss of blood supply to the area. Symptoms include:
- Paralysis below the level of injury
- Loss of pain and temperature sensation below the level of injury
- Intact sensations of touch, motion, position, and vibration.

The prognosis depends on the amount of damage. Surgical decompression may be done.

b. Central cord syndrome. This may be caused by hyperextension injuries or a lack of blood supply to the spinal cord. Central cord edema and/or hemorrhage can occur. As a result, there is a greater proportion of motor weakness in the upper extremities than in the lower.

c. Brown-Séquard syndrome. Penetrating injury may transect the cord from anterior to posterior on only one side, producing the following signs and symptoms:
- Ipsilateral paralysis below the lesion
- Ipsilateral loss of touch, pressure, vibration, and proprioception below the lesion
- Contralateral loss of pain and temperature sensation below the lesion.

J. Functional loss and expectations following spinal cord injury

The loss of function from spinal cord injuries depends on the segments involved and the extent of injury. Table 8-1 describes the lost functions and rehabilitative potential of patients with specific levels of spinal injuries.

TABLE 8-1

FUNCTIONAL LOSS AND EXPECTATIONS FOLLOWING SPINAL CORD INJURY

Level of injury	Functional loss	Functional expectation
Cervical (above C_5) Quadriplegia	Loss of motor and sensory function from neck and below. C_1 and C_2 injury is fatal. C_{3-5} can lead to respiratory paralysis. No bowel or bladder control	Total dependency. Ventilatory support
Cervical (C_5) Quadriplegia	Motor function lost below upper shoulders. Loss of sensation below clavicle. Sensation present in part of forearms. No innervation to intercostal muscles. No bowel or bladder control	Requires assistance in all activities. Possible ambulation in electric wheelchair. May feed self with special devices
Cervical (C_6) Quadriplegia	Motor function lost below shoulders and upper arms. More arm and thumb sensation than C_5; otherwise the same	Requires assistive devices for self-care activities. Electric wheelchair for ambulation. Assistance for transfer
Cervical (C_7) Quadriplegia	Intact motor function in shoulders, elbows, wrists, and part of hands. More sensation in arms and hands than C_6. Remainder of function loss same as C_5	Increased ability to perform activities of daily living. Ambulates in wheelchair with special handgrasps. Still requires assistance. May drive
Cervical (C_8) Quadriplegia	Able to control arms but may have some hand weakness. Sensation lost below chest. Remainder of function loss same as C_5	Able to use wheelchair and do pushups. Increased independence in activities of daily living. Self-catheterization ability and rectal stimulation
Thoracic (T_1-T_6) Paraplegia	Loss of motor ability and sensation below midchest. May have some intercostal muscle impairment. Loss of bowel and bladder control	May become completely independent in self-care. Able to work. Ambulation with wheelchair

Level of injury	Functional loss	Functional expectation
Thoracic (T_6-T_{12}) Paraplegia	Loss of motor ability and sensation below waist. Respiratory function intact, but no bowel or bladder control	Same as T_1-T_6, but with improved sitting balance
Lumbar (L_1-L_3) Paraplegia	Loss of motor function to pelvis and legs. Loss of sensation to lower abdomen and legs. No bowel or bladder control	Wheelchair independence. Some walking in long leg braces
Lumbosacral (L_4-S_1) Paraplegia (incomplete)	Some loss of motor function in hips, knees, and feet. Sensation intact in most of legs and feet. No bowel or bladder control	Ambulation with braces, canes, or crutches. Bowel evacuated by straining or manual removal. Bladder evacuated by straining and Credé
Sacral (S_2-S_4) Paraplegia (incomplete)	Loss of ankle plantar-flexors (S_2). Loss of sensation to part of legs (S_2) and perineum. Bowel and bladder function impaired initially	Ambulation normal. Bowel and bladder evacuation same as above

K. Initial assessment of the cord-injured patient

1. Physical assessment

First make sure there's a patent airway and the patient is breathing. Look at the skin color to detect cyanosis. Assess vital signs for evidence of spinal shock (hypotension, bradycardia, lowered body temperature) and hemorrhage (hypotension and tachycardia). Then perform a neurologic exam to establish a baseline, determine the level of the lesion, and detect the presence of head injury.

2. Gathering pertinent information

The following information is vital for appropriate management of the patient:

a. History of the accident. The history of the accident should include:
- Mechanism of injury
- Physical status after injury
- Treatment at accident site
- Mode of transportation to hospital.

b. Medical history. In addition to an account of the accident, it's important to know the following:
- Pre-existing diseases
- Use of drugs, alcohol, prescription medications
- Any known allergies
- Presence and extent of other injuries.

3. Diagnostic studies

a. Laboratory studies. Obtain the following baseline studies and evaluate for abnormalities:
- Electrolytes, glucose
- Hemoglobin and hematocrit
- Blood gases
- Coagulation studies
- Urinalysis
- Blood for type and cross-match.

b. Radiographic studies. X-rays should include anteroposterior and lateral spine films.

c. Myelogram. This study usually is performed after the patient has been stabilized.

4. Other measures

A Foley catheter is inserted to monitor urinary output. A nasogastric tube is usually inserted to prevent vomiting.

L. Medical management of the cord-injured patient

Medical goals during the acute phase include controlling edema of the spinal cord and reducing and immobilizing vertebral fractures if present. To control edema, corticosteroid therapy is begun with dexamethasone sodium phosphate (Decadron phosphate) or other steroid preparation. Restoring normal alignment with the use of skeletal traction may decompress the cord, relieve pain, and prevent further damage.

Surgery may be done in the acute phase in the hopes of preserving spinal cord function. Permanent surgical stabilization may be done after the acute phase if natural healing does not take place.

M. Problems and complications
1. Respiratory problems

An aggressive respiratory program is ordered to prevent atelectasis, infections, and respiratory failure.

2. Thrombophlebitis

Thrombophlebitis is a common complication that requires treatment with heparin or warfarin (Coumadin). Prophylactic administration of low-dose heparin may be ordered.

3. Orthostatic hypotension

The presence of orthostatic hypotension may require the administration of vasopressor drugs.

4. Autonomic hyperreflexia

Autonomic hyperreflexia is a serious emergency characterized by paroxysmal severe hypertension. Signs and symptoms include headache, flushing, profuse sweating, nausea, piloerection above the lesion level, and chest pain. These symptoms can lead to status epilepticus, stroke, and death.

Autonomic hyperreflexia is caused by reflex stimulation of the sympathetic nervous system by a noxious stimulus, usually a distended bladder, fecal impaction or decubitus ulcer. Immediate treatment includes placing the patient in an upright position, notifying the physician, and removal of the noxious stimulus. Drug therapy may include administration of hydralazine (Apresoline), diazoxide (Hyperstat), or ganglionic blocking agents to control blood pressure.

5. Spasticity

Spasticity, a problem that often occurs, may be treated by passive range of motion exercises and drug therapy with agents such as diazepam (Valium) or dantrolene (Dantrium). Surgery may be necessary.

6. Bladder atony

Atonic bladder is treated with insertion of a Foley catheter or an intermittent catheterization program. Care must be taken to prevent urinary infection. Prophylactic sulfa drugs may be ordered. Bladder training may eventually be necessary for neurogenic bladder.

7. Constipation

Prevention of constipation requires administration of stool softeners and milk of magnesia. Suppositories may be necessary. Occasionally an enema may be needed. In the rehabilitative phase, a bowel training program is begun.

N. Nursing assessment and management of the cord-injured patient

During the acute phase, observe for signs of respiratory impairment. Assess breath sounds and evaluate blood gases. Perform neurologic assessments frequently: level of consciousness, pupillary signs, eye movement, and motor, sensory, and cranial nerve function. Assess for signs of thrombophlebitis: redness, warmth, tenderness, and swelling. Evaluate bladder and bowel function daily.

After the patient becomes stabilized, include assessment for skin breakdown or pressure areas; observe urine output and characteristics and check for bladder distention.

In caring for the cord-injured patient your goals should include prevention of respiratory complications, thrombophlebitis, bladder overdistention and infection, skin breakdown, orthostatic hypotension, musculoskeletal deformities, and spasticity. Further responsibilities include promotion of proper hydration and nutrition, management of orthopedic equipment, maintaining bowel and bladder function, and emotional support of patient and family. Refer to Chapter 5 for general principles of nursing management.

O. Rehabilitation of the cord-injured patient

The rehabilitation process seeks to achieve the optimal level of function for the spinal-cord-injured patient. Helping him reach this goal involves all health team members. Much teaching and emotional support are needed. The bibliography at the end of this book provides sources of information on rehabilitation of the spinal-cord-injured patient.

QUIZ

1. While playing shortstop, Mr. J was hit in the head by a baseball and suffered a contusion of brain tissue. Keeping in mind the mechanisms of head injury, he probably sustained a:
   a. Contrecoup lesion
   b. Shearing lesion
   c. Coup lesion
   d. Distortion lesion

2. Ms. T was admitted to the hospital emergency department after a fall. Initially she experienced loss of consciousness, but was again alert and oriented on admission. While you are caring for her, her level of consciousness begins to decline. What type of head injury would you expect she sustained?
   a. Cerebral contusion
   b. Intracerebral hematoma
   c. Subdural hematoma
   d. Epidural hematoma

3. The primary consideration in initial management of a head-injured patient is:
   a. Evaluate level of consciousness
   b. Establish an airway
   c. Give oxygen
   d. Assess for hemorrhage

4. Which of the following is *not* true regarding the pathophysiology of spinal cord injury?
   a. Spinal cord injury is usually due to vertebral trauma
   b. Paralysis is most often the result of a torn spinal cord

c. The injury causes hemorrhage and necrosis of the spinal cord gray matter
   d. Trauma causes edema in spinal cord white matter
5. Which of the following are symptoms of spinal shock?
   a. Hypotension
   b. Hyperreflexia
   c. Loss of sensation below the injury level
   d. Spastic paralysis
6. Mr. P, a spinal-cord-injured patient, is experiencing signs and symptoms of left-sided paralysis—loss of touch, pressure, vibration, and proprioception—and right-sided loss of pain and temperature sensation. What type of partial cord injury is he likely to have?
   a. Central cord syndrome
   b. Anterior cord syndrome
   c. Brown-Séquard syndrome
   d. Posterior cord syndrome
7. Goals of management of the spinal-cord-injured patient in the acute phase include:
   a. Control of spinal cord edema
   b. Reduction and immobilization of injuries
   c. Prevention of autonomic hyperreflexia
   d. Prevention of acute seizure activity
8. Mr. B, a quadriplegic in the acute phase, suddenly develops severe hypertension. What actions would you carry out?
   a. Call the physician immediately
   b. Check for the presence of noxious stimuli
   c. Check for bladder distention or blockage of the indwelling catheter
   d. Decrease intravenous fluids
   e. Raise the patient's head

ANSWERS

1. c.   **5.** a, c.
2. d.   **6.** c.
3. b.   **7.** a, b.
4. b.   **8.** a, b, c, e.

CHAPTER

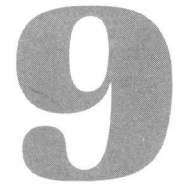

Tumors of the Central Nervous System

OBJECTIVES

After completing this chapter, you will be able to:

1. *Discuss the pathophysiology of brain and spinal tumors*
2. *Identify the signs and symptoms of brain and spinal tumors*
3. *Describe the types of brain tumors that affect adults*
4. *Identify the procedures utilized to diagnose tumors of the CNS*
5. *Discuss pre- and post-treatment nursing assessment*
6. *Discuss the classification of spinal cord tumors*
7. *Discuss nursing management goals for patients with brain and spinal cord tumors.*

A. Pathophysiology of brain tumors

This discussion will focus primarily on brain tumors in adults.

1. Incidence

Approximately 15,000 deaths occur each year in the United States from intracranial tumors—an incidence of primary brain tumors of 4.5/100,000. Peak incidence occurs in children and in the fifth decade of life. The incidence of primary brain tumors is highest in white males and lowest in nonwhite females.

2. Etiology

Although the exact cause of brain tumors is unknown, the relationships between brain tumors and various factors are being investigated. These supposed risk factors include exposure to chemical carcinogens, familial predisposition, exposure to certain drugs, immunosuppression, infectious agents, radiation, and trauma.

Unfortunately, there is little evidence linking these factors with brain tumors.

3. Tumor growth

Tumor cells typically form a mass that grows until it meets an obstacle. Tumor cells can also infiltrate brain tissue. Masses grow primarily by cell reproduction, and secondarily by invading and destroying surrounding tissue through hemorrhage, ischemia, and necrosis. Compression of brain tissue usually results in cerebral edema. Edema, together with increased tumor size, eventually produces signs of increased intracranial pressure (see Chapter 4).

Most primary brain tumors are located in the supratentorial region. The continuing pressure causes herniation of brain tissue downward. Without treatment, the brain will herniate down through the foramen magnum and death due to compression of vital centers will result.

Functional deficits are due to compression, infiltration, and edema formation. Specific focal neurologic deficits depend on the area of the brain invaded by tumor cells. Tumors near or within the ventricles or subarachnoid space can cause obstruction of the flow of cerebrospinal fluid and resulting hydrocephalus. Tumors of or near the pituitary gland may cause endocrine imbalances.

Cerebral compression or edema may produce seizures. Seizures begin in the gray matter of the brain. If they occur, the tumor will be found on the brain surface.

B. Signs and symptoms of brain tumors

Brain tumor symptoms depend on the type of tumor, its location, and its rate of growth. Some tumors grow slowly and present no symptoms until they are very large. Tumors in the medulla or other vital areas cause symptoms that appear earlier, because they interfere with vital functions such as breathing and blood pressure.

Common signs and symptoms of brain tumors are the following:
- Increased intracranial pressure: decreased level of consciousness (usually the earliest sign), pupillary changes, decreased eye movement, loss of motor or sensory function, alterations in respirations, alterations in vital signs
- Seizure activity
- Headache
- Vomiting
- Papilledema
- Endocrine imbalance associated with pituitary dysfunction
- Personality and intellectual changes
- Motor dysfunctions
- Sensory dysfunctions
- Loss of coordination
- Cranial nerve dysfunction.

C. Classification of brain tumors

There is no universally accepted classification of brain tumors. Following are several in use:

1. Primary versus secondary tumors

Primary brain tumors arise from nerve tissue; secondary tumors are metastases from other sites in the body.

2. Malignant versus benign tumors

Brain tumors that are considered histologically benign can still be serious if they cannot be removed and continue to grow, increasing intracranial pressure or impairing vital functions.

3. Supratentorial versus infratentorial

This distinction is mostly of anatomical significance.

4. Childhood- versus adult-onset tumors

Certain types of brain tumors are more common in children; others, in adults.

5. Cellular and anatomic origin

This system, based on the cellular histology and anatomic origin of the tumor cells, is the most familiar, and is used in the rest of this chapter.

The following tumors are those that most often affect adults.

a. Astrocytoma (grades I and II). Usually found in the cerebral hemispheres, these tumors are characterized according to whether the cells are well differentiated (grade I) or less differentiated (grade II). Neurologic deficits depend on the location of the tumor. This type of astrocytoma rarely is completely removed, and radiation is used only with the grade II type. The survival rate is 6 to 10 years.

b. Astrocytoma (grades III and IV). These tumors are also called glioblastoma multiforme, and are highly malignant and rapidly growing. They are most prevalent in men aged 40 to 60. These tumors are frequently found in the white matter of the cerebral hemispheres, with symptoms dependent on location. Usually surgery for resection and decompression is performed, followed by radiation and chemotherapy. The survival rate is less than 2 years.

c. Oligodendroglioma. This is a slowly growing tumor of the cerebral hemispheres. It is most common in the 20- to 40-year age group. Symptoms depend on the location of the tumor, but seizures are often the first symptom. Radiation is used if surgery is unsuccessful in removing the entire tumor.

d. Meningioma. A meningioma is an encapsulated, slowly growing tumor of arachnoid granulations. It invades the skull and dura, but rarely the cerebral tissue. Rather, symptoms are due to compression and displacement of the surrounding area and depend on location. Meningiomas most frequently affect middle-aged women. Radiation is used if the tumor is not completely removed by surgery.

e. Acoustic neuroma. This benign tumor arises from the vestibular branch of cranial nerve VIII. As it grows, it may involve cranial nerves VII, IX, X, and V, causing facial asymmetry, weakness, loss of sensation, and difficulty swallowing and speaking. In the earlier stages, tinnitus, hearing loss, and dizziness are common symptoms. Surgery is the usual treatment. If the tumor is completely removed, the prognosis is excellent.

f. Hemangioblastoma. A hemangioblastoma is a vascular, slowly growing tumor found in the cerebellum, and sometimes in the medulla or cerebrum. Patients may complain of headache and other symptoms of increased intracranial pressure, loss of coordination, and ataxia – the latter two due to cerebellar involvement. Hemangioblastomas are usually curable by surgery and radiation.

g. Pituitary tumors. These slow growing, encapsulated, benign tumors usually arise in the anterior lobe of the pituitary gland, although both lobes can be affected. *Chromophobic* pituitary adenomas are the most common type of pituitary tumor. Symptoms include hypopituitarism, visual field defects, and headaches. *Basophilic* adenomas secrete adrenocorticotropic hormones and produce Cushing's syndrome. *Eosinophilic* adenomas secrete growth hormones and can produce gigantism before puberty and acromegaly after puberty. Treatment may include a combination of surgery (transsphenoidal hypophysectomy), radiation, and drug therapy. The prognosis is good.

h. Metastatic brain tumors. These tumors have metastasized from carcinomas in other parts of the body and can appear at multiple sites in the brain. The lungs, breasts, kidneys, thyroid, and gastrointestinal tract are the most common sources. Symptoms depend on the location of the tumor. Surgery may be done. Prognosis is poor.

D. Diagnosis of brain tumors

In conjunction with the history and physical, diagnostic studies that can help in determining the presence of a brain tumor include:
- Skull films — may reveal erosion of bone, pineal gland shifts, and calcifications of the tumor
- CT scan — can determine presence, size, and location of a tumor
- Visual field and funduscopic examination — can help localize the tumor and reveal presence of papilledema, respectively
- Electroencephalogram — found in about 75 percent of patients with tumors, abnormal EEG tracings can also help locate tumor
- Brain scan — shows size and location of tumor; since tumor cells take up more radioisotope than surrounding normal cells
- Lumbar puncture — measures CFS pressure and may reveal cancerous cells; should not be done in patients with increased intracranial pressure
- Cerebral angiography — can demonstrate distortion of blood vessels or abnormal vascularity and thus help diagnose tumor type
- Echoencephalography — can identify a shift in midline structures due to a tumor
- Endocrine studies — can help detect pituitary tumors.

E. Nursing assessment of the patient with a brain tumor

Prior to diagnosis, your primary responsibilities include teaching your patient about the diagnostic procedures he will undergo and giving emotional support.

After diagnosis, treatment — surgery, chemotherapy, and/or radiation — will be planned. Provide your patient with an environment that's supportive and conducive to questioning and planning realistically for the future. Because all cancer treatments tend to be debilitating, nursing assessment becomes an especially important aspect of therapy.

1. Surgery

Surgery is performed to diagnose the tumor exactly, remove it if possible, or resect enough tissue to relieve compression and increased intracranial pressure. Most brain surgery involves craniotomy.

a. Preoperative assessment. Discuss what the patient knows about his surgery, answer questions, clarify misconceptions, and explain what the patient can expect postoperatively – including shaving of his head in the area to be cut.

Before surgery, a neurologic assessment provides a baseline for postoperative monitoring and evaluation. Complete your hospital's preoperative checklist. Be sure to examine the patient's blood studies, EEG, and chest film evaluation for any abnormalities that would affect surgery. Preoperative preparation – including withholding of food – is the same as for any other kind of surgery.

b. Postoperative assessment. Your tasks at this stage include assessing neurologic status, observing for and preventing complications, providing supportive care, and aiding in rehabilitation (see chapter 5 for specifics).

Assess neurologic status as often as the patient's condition requires, looking especially for signs of increased intracranial pressure. Respiratory assessment, as always, is an important part of postoperative care. Fever in the first 24 to 48 hours is often respiratory in origin. Possible respiratory complications include pneumonia, atelectasis, emboli, and pulmonary emboli.

Auscultate for the return of bowel sounds. Evaluate the ability to swallow before each oral feeding, and check for alterations in bowel elimination.

Assess urinary output and specific gravity, especially if the pituitary was involved. If transient diabetes insipidus occurs, it may be treated with intramuscular injection of vasopressin (Pitressin) and intravenous replacement of fluid and electrolytes. Also evaluate the urine for symptoms of infection.

Observe the head dressings for drainage, which is to be expected if a drain is in place. Change or reinforce dressings as necessary to prevent infection.

Assess for the presence of a corneal reflex, periorbital edema, or inability to close the eye completely. You may need to institute special eye care (see Chapter 5).

Assess body temperature frequently. Hyperthermia is a common postoperative complication that can be due to atelectasis, infection, or irritation to hypothalamic centers.

Hypovolemic shock may be recognized by tachycardia, hypotension, rapid respirations, restlessness, decreased urine output, and cool skin. Assessing for this complication requires frequent observations of blood pressure, pulse, respirations, mentation, urine output, skin temperature, and central venous pressure. Treatment includes fluid expanders and vasodilating drugs.

Increased intracranial pressure can be caused by cerebral edema, hemorrhage, meningitis, or surgical trauma. Assessing level of consciousness is the primary method of evaluating intracranial pressure (see Chapter 4).

Seizures sometimes occur following cranial surgery, so observe for evidence of seizure activity and institute seizure precautions. Following surgery, patients usually receive prophylactic phenytoin (Dilantin).

Cerebrospinal fluid leaks from the wound, nose (rhinorrhea), or ear (otorrhea) may result. If the drainage is bloody, observe for a clear ring around the blood on the dressing or towel. The ring indicates CSF. You can make sure that clear drainage is CSF by testing it for glucose (Dextrostix). Nose blowing, suctioning, and positive pressure breathing are contraindicated if the patient has rhinorrhea. Antibiotics may be ordered. Additional surgery may be needed to repair the leak.

Hydrocephalus can result from edema or bleeding, most often after posterior fossa surgery. Surgical shunting is usually done.

Assess cranial nerve function, since deficits can occur following surgery. Some of the more common complications in this area include visual field deficits, diplopia, and loss of the gag reflex and ability to swallow.

Evaluate the patient's ability to communicate. Aphasia can occur after surgery, and the exact type should be determined. Refer to Chapter 5 for management of communication deficits.

Finally, psychosocial needs are a vital part of postoperative assessment. Support the patient and family as they try to deal with possible deficits. Provide explanations for all that is occurring. Use of scarves to cover a woman's head may help her deal with her temporary baldness. Your role in providing information and support to the family is essential during the recovery period.

2. Chemotherapy

Chemotherapy may be used along with surgery and/or radiation therapy. The regimen depends on the tumor's type and location and the patient's tolerance.

You can assess the patient's tolerance by looking for side effects of these drugs: nausea, vomiting, diarrhea, stomatitis, anorexia, hair loss, and bone marrow depression. Be sure the patient knows they may occur.

You may be able to control nausea and vomiting by giving an antiemetic and a light meal before chemotherapy. Ice chips and ginger ale occasionally can relieve these symptoms. To counteract anorexia, offer the patient the foods he likes best, in small feedings. You may relieve diarrhea with an antidiarrheal agent.

Stomatitis requires good oral hygiene and application of a topical anesthetic to relieve pain. The patient should avoid foods that irritate the mucous membranes.

Encourage patients who develop alopecia to cover their heads with wigs, scarves, or turbans. Make sure they understand their hair will grow back once chemotherapy ends.

Look for signs of infection and hemorrhage; they may indicate bone marrow depression. If blood counts reveal decreases in white cells and platelets, replacement of these components may be necessary.

3. Radiation therapy

The goal of radiation therapy is to destroy radiosensitive cancer cells without destroying healthy cells. The amount of exposure depends on the type of tumor, the location, its response to radiation, and its level of tolerance. Radiation may be used instead of or in addition to surgery when the tumor cannot be excised completely. Radiation may improve the patient's condition, but it may cause radiation edema, elevate intracranial pressure, and worsen symptoms.

Provide the patient and family with information about the radiation therapy department and what to expect. As with chemotherapy, nausea, vomiting, diarrhea, anorexia, and bone marrow depression can occur. Assess skin for sensitivity and protect it as necessary, but do not apply any substance to it. Do not wash off skin markings. Reassure the patient that the symptoms will stop after therapy ends.

F. Pathophysiology of spinal cord tumors

Spinal cord tumors are rare, comprising only about 0.5 to 1 percent of all tumors, and the majority are usually benign. They are more common in the 20- to 60-year age group, rarely occurring before the age of 10. Males and females seem to be affected equally.

Spinal cord tumors are rarely fatal but can cause severe disabilities. Recovery time varies, depending on tumor type and success of treatment.

Spinal cord tumors affect the cord more by compression than by invasion. Direct pressure on the cord can result in:
- Compression of spinal arteries and veins
- Interference with conduction of spinal roots and tracts
- Obstruction of cerebrospinal fluid flow
- Edema formation below the compression.

The spinal cord can accommodate slowly growing soft tumors (e.g., meningioma) with minimal resulting deficits. However, fast growing tumors, such as malignant or metastatic lesions, are poorly tolerated and deficits will occur rapidly. With movement, hard tumors can cause cord contusion, ischemia, and irreversible cord damage.

G. Classification of spinal cord tumors

1. Intradural tumors

These are located within or under the dura. There are two types:

Intramedullary tumors, which originate within the spinal cord, usually ependymomas and astrocytomas and extramedullary tumors, which originate within the dura mater, but outside the spinal cord itself. Neurinomas and meningiomas are the predominant types.

2. Extradural tumors

These tumors originate between the periosteum and the dura, and arise from the bones of the spinal column. A large percentage are metastatic, meningiomas, and neurinomas.

3. Extravertebral tumors

These are located partly within and outside the cord.

H. Signs and symptoms of spinal cord tumors

1. Pain

This is the most common complaint of patients with spinal cord tumors, and may sometimes be the only symptom. Some common types of pain include:

a. Local neck or back pain. This usually has a gradual onset but can occur suddenly. It is often aggravated by the Valsalva maneuver or by lying in bed, which stretches the spinal nerves.

b. Radicular pain. This type of pain traverses the distribution of the nerve root. Caused by irritation, compression, or tension on the nerve root, it is aggravated by movement, coughing, sneezing, or straining.

2. Motor disturbance

This disturbance presents as weakness and functional loss below the level of the lesion. Early symptoms include clumsiness, spasticity, and hyperactive reflexes, all of which arise from involvement of the corticospinal tract.

3. Sensory disturbances

The most common symptoms of sensory disturbance are loss of pain and temperature sensation, evidenced by early symptoms of numbness, tingling, or coldness. Later symptoms include loss of touch, vibration, and position sense.

A combination of motor and sensory symptoms — the Brown-Séquard syndrome — can arise from a lesion on the lateral portion of the spinal cord (see Chapter 8).

4. Sphincter disturbances

Bladder control is lost before bowel control. Symptoms include difficulty in evacuation, retention, constipation, incontinence, and impotence.

5. Papilledema

Papilledema is associated with lesions in the thoracic and lumbar regions. It is caused by increased intracranial pressure due to increased CSF volume and/or increased CSF pressure due to obstruction of flow.

I. Diagnosis of spinal cord tumors

To arrive at an accurate diagnosis of spinal cord tumor is a challenging process, because symptoms are often similar to those of such diseases as multiple sclerosis, amyotrophic lateral sclerosis, arachnoiditis, syringomyelia, hysteria, spondylosis, and herniated discs.

After a detailed history and physical, including a neurologic exam, the diagnosis is confirmed using some or all of the following procedures:

- Spinal X-ray — will reveal lesions affecting the vertebral column
- Lumbar puncture — may reveal elevated protein levels or tumor cells in CSF; Queckenstedt's sign (failure of CSF flow to increase when jugular veins are compressed) or a dry tap also indicates blockage
- Myelography — the most important test; demonstrates the level and completeness of spinal block and may outline

the tumor if the subarachnoid space is incompletely blocked
- CT scan – may reveal the presence of an extramedullary tumor
- Electromyography – often helpful in differential diagnosis.

J. Medical management of the patient with a spinal cord tumor

Medical management consists of controlling the symptoms of the tumor, and, when possible, surgical excision with or without radiation and chemotherapy. The specific treatment depends on the type of tumor, its location, and responsiveness. In general, extradural and intradural extramedullary tumors can be completely removed. Intramedullary tumors are not as easily removed, but the attempt is made. Metastatic lesions are managed with radiation, chemotherapy, and pain control. Some tumors respond to radiation after surgery better than others.

At the time of diagnosis, corticosteroids are usually administered to decrease edema. Maalox and cimetidine (Tagamet) are given in conjunction with steroids to decrease gastric irritation.

K. Nursing care of the patient with a spinal cord tumor

Obtain baseline data on the patient's neurologic function, respiratory function, vital signs, and sphincter control.

The neurologic evaluation should include testing the patient's motor function by assessing movement, muscle strength, muscle tone, coordination, and deep tendon reflexes. Test for sensory function by assessing the presence of light touch, pain, position sense, and temperature sensation.

Evaluate the patient's respiratory function by assessing breathing rate, amplitude, and rhythm. Auscultate for breath sounds and observe the symmetry of chest movement. Monitor arterial blood gases.

Assess vital signs. Hypotension might occur if vasomotor tone has been affected.

Evaluate sphincter control. Note urine output and frequency of voiding. Observe for signs of urinary infection and obtain a urine culture if warranted. Check for bladder and abdominal distention. Auscultate for bowel sounds.

Assess the patient's complaints of pain. Medicate and provide comfort measures as necessary. Evaluate his skin condition frequently, especially if sensation is affected.

As with brain surgery, it's important to provide basic hygienic and skin care, maintain proper positioning, promote adequate circulation, prevent musculoskeletal complications, provide proper nutrition, and promote safety.

Nursing management will depend on the extent and type of deficits. Your goals are preventing respiratory difficulties, promoting mobility, maintaining skin integrity, managing bowel and bladder difficulties, and teaching the patient to deal with his deficits.

QUIZ

1. Brain tumors _____ and _____ surrounding tissue.

2. Brain tumors are most often located in the
   a. Frontal lobe
   b. Supratentorial region
   c. Infratentorial region
   d. Diencephalon

3. Which of the following is the earliest sign of increasing intracranial pressure?
   a. Respiratory changes
   b. Alterations in vital signs
   c. Headache
   d. Changes in level of consciousness

4. Primary brain tumors arise from _____ tissue.

5. Astrocytoma grade IV is also called _____
   _____.

6. Which of the following should you include in your assessment of the patient following craniotomy?
   a. Increasing intracranial pressure
   b. Drainage from the wound
   c. Hyperthermia
   d. Bowel sounds
   e. Urinary output
   f. All of the above

7. Complications of cranial surgery include:
   a. Seizures
   b. Hyperthermia
   c. Hydrocephalus
   d. Diabetes insipidus
   e. All of the above

8. To help prevent nausea and vomiting after chemotherapy, you could:
   a. Maintain the patient on IV therapy
   b. Offer ice chips or ginger ale
   c. Administer an antiemetic before drug administration
   d. Decrease oral intake prior to drug administration

9. A spinal cord tumor affects the cord by _____
   _____.

10. The most common complaint that occurs with spinal cord tumors is _____.

11. The most important procedure in the diagnosis of spinal cord tumors is _____.

12. Your assessment of the patient with a spinal cord tumor should always include:
    a. Evaluating deep tendon reflexes
    b. Assessing respiratory function
    c. Evaluating cranial nerve function
    d. Assessing mental function

ANSWERS

1. Compress; infiltrate.
2. **b.**
3. **d.**
4. Nerve.
5. Glioblastoma multiforme.
6. **f.**
7. **e.**
8. **b, c, d.**
9. Compressing it.
10. Pain.
11. Myelogram.
12. **a, b.**

CHAPTER 10

Degenerative Diseases

OBJECTIVES

After completing this chapter, you will be able to:

1. Discuss the pathophysiology, signs, and symptoms of multiple sclerosis
2. Describe the pathophysiology, categories, classification, and signs and symptoms of Parkinson's disease
3. Discuss amyotrophic lateral sclerosis, including its pathophysiology, signs, and symptoms
4. Discuss medical management and nursing assessment and interventions in these degenerative diseases.

A. Multiple sclerosis

1. Description

Multiple sclerosis (MS) is a chronic, degenerative disease of the central nervous system that destroys myelin in the white matter of the brain and spinal cord.

2. Etiology

The exact cause of MS is unknown, but some theories link it to viral infections, while others suggest a possible deficiency in the immune system. Still another hypothesis is that the patient produces antibodies against his own nervous tissue.

3. Incidence

More than 500,000 people in the United States have MS. It occurs most frequently between the ages of 20 and 40, with women affected slightly more often than men. There is no proof that it is a genetic disease, but it does appear to be familial. MS is also more common in colder northern climates than in subtropical and tropical climates.

4. Pathophysiology

MS causes demyelination in scattered areas of the white matter of the brain and spinal cord. Initially there is breakdown of the myelin sheath but the nerve remains intact. The disease process has periods of remission, during which the affected myelin sheaths may regenerate, causing symptoms to disappear.

Eventually, however, the sclerotic tissue is replaced by scar tissue called plaque. The nerve fibers can also degenerate with scar tissue formation, causing permanent disability.

5. Signs and symptoms

The scattered involvement of the CNS produces a wide variety of symptoms in the MS patient. The following are most commonly encountered:
- Motor—weakness, incoordination, tremor, ataxia, paralysis, stiffness, spasticity
- Sensory—numbness, tingling, dizziness, sensory loss; occasionally, pain due to spasms

- Visual – blurred vision, diplopia, nystagmus, scotomas, pain on eye movement
- Speech impairment – dysarthria with slurred speech or scanning speech (slow speech with pauses between syllables)
- Impaired elimination – urinary urgency, frequency, retention, incontinence; bowel incontinence or constipation
- Sexual problems – impotence in men; loss of vaginal sensation in women
- Mental and behavioral changes – emotional lability, euphoria, depression, irritability, poor judgment; later in disease course, depression, confusion, memory deficits, disorientation
- Other symptoms – fatigue, lassitude, heat intolerance.

6. Disease progression

As with its symptoms, the course of MS can vary widely. In some patients there may be few exacerbations interspersed with long periods of remission. In others, the disease may produce acute exacerbations that leave permanent deficits after each attack. The irregular nature of MS makes it impossible to predict when the next attack will occur.

7. Precipitating factors

Infections, trauma, and pregnancy are all factors known to precipitate multiple sclerosis. Exacerbations may be caused by stress, fatigue, temperature extremes, menstruation, or poor health.

8. Diagnosis

Because there is no specific diagnostic test for MS, the diagnosis is usually made on the basis of the patient's history and neurologic deficits in an exacerbation-remission cycle. Tests that can suggest, though not diagnose, MS include:

a. Cerebrospinal fluid analysis. About 75 percent of MS patients have elevated CSF gamma globulins in the later stages of the disease. Electrophoresis of CSF may produce oligoclonal bands that represent an immunoglobulin response. Oligoclonal banding is increased in 80 percent of MS patients.

b. Visual evoked response. When optic neuritis is not present, delays in conduction speed may help support the diagnosis of MS.

c. Raising nerve temperature. When body temperature is raised by exposure to heat, the affected nerves may stop transmitting impulses, producing symptoms.

d. CT scan. About 20 percent of MS patients have a lesion that may be visualized by this method.

9. Medical management of the patient with MS

Treatment is directed toward shortening the duration of acute exacerbations, alleviating symptoms, and providing support.

Drug therapy may include the use of adrenocorticotropin (ACTH) or prednisone to help shorten an exacerbation. Some believe a low-fat diet may alter the progressive course of the disease. Dorsal column stimulation may be used to decrease pain and spasticity. Physical therapy may also help reduce spasticity.

10. Nursing assessment of the patient with MS

A patient with multiple sclerosis is most often seen in an acute care facility during an acute exacerbation, sometimes for treatment of a complication or an unrelated problem. During hospitalization, your main goal should be to help him reach his highest functional level. The following discussion includes problems you may encounter, but remember that each patient's needs are individual.

a. Planning care. Planning your patient's care requires a thorough assessment. Obtain a history of the course of his disease. Do a thorough neurologic assessment to establish the extent of involvement. Determine what the patient can and can't do for himself. Be sure your plan of care allows the patient to continue his independent activities.

b. Psychological needs. A patient not yet diagnosed may require your support and teaching to help him deal with fear of the diagnostic outcome. Once a diagnosis is made, the patient may deny or grieve. Your support is necessary to help him understand and accept his diagnosis. Help the patient maintain control by allowing him to participate in planning care and setting goals. A patient who has had MS for some time still needs your support to continue to cope with any limitations.

c. Sensory problems. Sensory involvement may include diminished temperature or touch perception, diminished position sense, paresthesia, and pain. Educate the patient to test bath water with an unaffected part, use potholders when cooking, and wear gloves when the weather is cold. Painful sensations may be treated with carbamazepine (Tegretol). Teach the patient to watch what he does, to make up for lack of position and touch sensation.

d. Motor difficulties. Evaluate the patient's motor involvement. Physical therapy with active and passive exercises may be instituted. Gait training may be necessary. Assistive devices such as braces, walkers, and canes may help improve ambulation. Bed rest during exacerbation may be necessary since fatigue can worsen symptoms. And, ;when possible, rest periods and exercise should be included in the care plan.

e. Spasticity. Drugs such as diazepam (Valium), baclofen (Lioresal), and dantrolene (Dantrium) may be prescribed to decrease spasticity. Range of motion exercises are necessary. Night splinting of the involved parts is useful. Cold application to the extremity may relax spasticity.

f. Ataxia. Ataxia of the lower extremities may affect ambulation. Stability can be improved by widening the gait or utilizing a cane or a walker. Upper extremity ataxia may require the use of special eating utensils. Patients with head tremor may require a collar or neck brace.

g. Visual difficulties. Patients with diplopia may require the use of an eye patch or eyeglass occluder. Reassure the patient that visual symptoms usually remit and permanent blindness is rare.

h. Speech difficulties. Dysarthria may require the skill of a speech therapist if communication abilities are severely impaired. Be sure to take the time to listen carefully to what the patient says.

i. Bladder dysfunction. Bladder problems can affect activities of daily living and result in urinary tract infections. Assess for the presence of bladder dysfunction. Patients who have high residual urine levels require increased fluid intake. Assess for signs of urinary tract infection and teach them to the patient so he can detect and report them early.

Patients with frequency and urgency may need anticholinergic drugs to decrease bladder spasticity. Baclofen or bethanechol (Urecholine) may also be necessary.

A bladder training program utilizing such techniques as the Credé maneuver and intermittent catheterization may need to be instituted. The patient can be taught to catheterize himself, or a family member can be taught. Every effort should be made to keep the patient dry and infection-free. Use of indwelling catheters should be avoided.

j. Bowel dysfunction. Incontinence and constipation are the major bowel problems. Bowel programs should include adequate fluid intake and high-roughage foods. Occasionally stool softeners, laxatives, or suppositories are helpful.

k. Psychosexual problems. Patients with MS do marry. However, if impotence or decreased vaginal sensation occurs, alternative sexual practices may need to be discussed. Encourage patients to articulate these problems. Having children is a serious decision—and may well be unwise if the patient's prognosis is poor. Counseling may be helpful for psychological and sexual problems, so making appropriate referrals is an important nursing task.

Sexual activity may be hampered by bowel and bladder dysfunction. Recommend emptying the bowel and bladder beforehand.

l. Problems of immobility. Patients who are inactive require more basic nursing care. Respiratory infection is a common problem and can be prevented by coughing and deep breathing. Teach the patient to avoid crowds. Discourage smoking.

Skin care should include turning, massage, and keeping the skin dry and clean. Patients in wheelchairs should be taught to shift position frequently. Special mattresses, sheepskin, silicone pads, heel and elbow pads, and similar aids should be utilized. Avoid the use of hot pads and hot baths. Range of motion exercises and antiembolic stockings are necessary for immobile patients. Refer to Chapter 5 for further information on management of mobility problems.

m. Economic issues. It isn't unusual for financial concerns to become a major issue. Here a social worker can be helpful. The National Multiple Sclerosis Society also provides many services, and the Bureau of Vocational Rehabilitation can help with vocational needs.

B. Parkinson's disease
1. Description
Parkinson's disease is a chronic degenerative disease of the basal ganglia that results in decreased production and storage of dopamine.

2. Incidence
The disease primarily affects those in their 50s and 60s, men slightly more often than women.

3. Causative agent
As with many degenerative diseases, the cause of Parkinson's disease is unknown. There are theories that it may result from an accelerated aging process, a virus, or an inherited genetic defect.

4. Etiologic categories
- Idiopathic – includes most of those currently affected
- Postencephalitic – affects survivors of the 1916-1926 encephalitis epidemic
- Drug-induced (pseudoparkinsonism) – caused by certain drugs such as phenothiazines and *Rauwolfia* alkaloids (reserpine), and is reversible when the drug is stopped.

5. Classification
- Stage I – mild, unilateral involvement
- Stage II – bilateral involvement, minimal disability
- Stage III – impaired postural and righting reflexes; mild to moderate disability
- Stage IV – fully developed, severe disease; significant disability
- Stage V – confinement to bed or wheelchair.

6. Pathophysiology

The degenerative changes of Parkinson's disease cause loss of neurons and the dopamine-rich cells of the substantia nigra. The inhibitory effect of dopamine is lost and the excitatory mechanisms are unopposed. Cell degeneration affects the extrapyramidal tracts, semiautomatic functions, and coordinated movements.

7. Signs and symptoms

Symptoms develop slowly and are progressive. They include:
- A masklike, expressionless face, with decreased blinking
- Bradykinesia (slowness of movement)
- Change in posture – trunk stooped forward; forearms semiflexed; shuffling gait
- Fatigue, weakness
- Muscle rigidity and cramps
- Tremors that appear at rest; "pill-rolling" movement of hands
- Restlessness
- Mental depression
- Others: drooling, dysphagia, weak voice, increased perspiration, oily skin, constipation, and urinary hesitation and frequency.

8. Diagnosis

Diagnosis is based on signs and symptoms, and is difficult to make in the early stages of the disease.

9. Medical management of the patient with Parkinson's disease

Therapy is directed toward control or relief of symptoms, primarily with drugs.

L-Dopa is the most important antiparkinsonian drug. This drug is converted into dopamine in the basal ganglia, thereby elevating dopamine levels and relieving symptoms. Because it is also converted to dopamine in the peripheral tissues, it can cause adverse reactions (see Appendix). Long-term use of L-dopa can result in the "on-off" phenomenon, a temporary worsening of symptoms that can last several hours and is treated by spreading out the daily dosage. Abnormal involuntary movements of the face, tongue, mouth, and head can occur. Lowering the dosage may lessen this effect. Occasionally a patient may stop responding to L-dopa. If this occurs, the patient may be given a short holiday from the drug.

Carbidopa, a dopa decarboxylase inhibitor, is often given with L-dopa as Sinemet (see Appendix) to prevent conversion of L-dopa to dopamine in peripheral tissues, thereby decreasing L-dopa's side effects.

Amantadine (Symmetrel), an antiviral medication, may also relieve symptoms. Although not as effective as L-dopa, it has fewer side effects (see Appendix).

Anticholinergic and antihistaminic agents may be utilized together to block the central cholinergic excitatory pathways and decrease the reuptake of dopamine in to presynaptic nerve endings. They are effective with mild parkinsonism. The more commonly used agents in this category and dosages can be found in Table 10-1.

TABLE 10-1

ANTICHOLINERGIC/ANTIHISTAMINIC DRUGS USED TO TREAT PARKINSON'S DISEASE

Drug	*Usual dosage*
Trihexyphenidyl (Artane)	6-10 mg/day
Biperiden (Akineton)	2 mg tid or qid
Cycrimine (Pagitane)	1.25-5 mg tid or qid
Procyclidine (Kemadrin)	4-5 mg tid or qid
Benztropine (Cogentin)	1-2 mg/day
Diphenhydramine (Benadryl)	50 mg tid or qid
Chlorphenoxamine (Phenoxene)	50-100 mg tid or qid
Orphenadrine (Disipal)	50 mg tid

10. Nursing assessment of the patient with Parkinson's disease

The patient with Parkinson's disease is usually seen in the acute care setting for diagnosis, adjustment of drug dosages, or treatment of an unrelated illness. You should take care to detect and fulfill the following specific needs:

a. Mobility. Observe the patient's posture, gait, and balance. Assess his ability to move from bed to chair. Evaluate the need for mobility aids like a walker or three-legged cane. An overhead trapeze may be helpful. Be sure the patient stands close to a chair before sitting. Bed rails must be elevated when the patient is in bed.

Help the patient maintain his level of mobility while hospitalized. Ambulation is important; teach the patient to use a wide-based stance if necessary. Avoid prolonged sitting, which can cause edema. Perform range of motion exercises to prevent contractures and stiffness.

Discuss the home environment. Scatter rugs should be removed. Wall handles in bathrooms should be added, if necessary. A rocking chair at home may stimulate circulation.

b. Nutritional needs. Evaluate the patient's eating habits and physical problems that can affect nutrition. Monitor the patient's weight daily. If the patient has difficulty swallowing, a soft, ground, or pureed diet in six small feedings may be better tolerated than the ordinary three large daily meals. Food may need to be cut for the patient. If possible, consult a dietitian. The patient may have trouble swallowing pills; tablets may need to be crushed or capsules opened.

At home the patient or family may need to prepare food with a blender. If the patient eats slowly, an electric warming tray can keep his food warm.

c. Elimination. Assess the patient's normal bowel habits. Parkinson's patients are prone to constipation. Encourage a diet of adequate fluid and fruit. Stool softeners, mild laxatives, or suppositories may be needed. Avoid frequent use of enemas

Assess for urinary hesitation and frequency. Incontinence of urine may be a problem. Evaluate the cause; it may be as simple as inability to reach the bathroom fast enough. If so, keep a urinal or bedpan within easy reach. A bedside commode may be helpful. Offer the bedpan or urinal frequently, or help the patient to the bathroom regularly.

d. Hygienic needs. The skin tends to be oily, and excessive perspiration may be a problem. A daily bath is necessary, with perhaps partial bathing in afternoon and evening. Frequent linen changes may be needed. Use deodorants.

e. Respiratory needs. Evaluate the patient's respiratory status. Teach him to cough and deep breathe. If he is on bed rest or tends to be fairly immobile, chest physical therapy and suctioning may be necessary.

f. Circulatory needs. If the patient is experiencing orthostatic hypotension or has decreased mobility, elastic stockings are a necessity. Explain to the patient that he should change positions slowly.

g. Maintaining independence. Assess the patient's ability to perform activities of daily living. Encourage him to do as much for himself as possible. Allow extra time for tasks, since he may do them slowly. Avoid rushing him.

At home, the patient can wear clothing with zippers or Velcro fasteners instead of buttons or snaps. He should wear slip-on shoes rather than ones with laces. He may need a raised toilet seat. Consult an occupational therapist to assist the patient in learning new techniques of caring for himself and to provide mechanical aids if needed.

h. Communication needs. The patient's voice may become soft and slow with slurred speech. Also, writing may be difficult. Encourage the patient to sing or read aloud for practice and to speak loudly. Take time to listen to the patient. Consult a speech therapist if one is available.

i. Emotional needs. Both the patient and the family need your support and encouragement. Frustration and mental depression are common. His symptoms may cause the patient to withdraw from social contact. Stress the patient's abilities, not his disabilities. Discuss his symptoms and help him and his family members accept them without embarrassment. Often an understanding family or significant other can do much to help the patient cope with his problems. However, referral to a psychiatric nurse specialist or psychiatrist may be necessary.

j. Patient and family education. The patient and family should gain a realistic understanding of the disease and its treatment. Drug education is of prime importance.

The patient taking L-dopa (Larodopa) or carbidopa-levodopa requires an explanation of the drug, its dosage, and its side effects. Encourage him to control his intake of high-protein foods, since large amounts of protein can block L-dopa's effect. To prevent nausea, L-dopa should be taken with meals. Orthostatic hypotension, common in the early months of therapy, can be counteracted as explained earlier.

Teach the patient about the early signs of overdosage, which include muscle twitching and intermittent winking. If he has been on long-term L-dopa therapy, he should be aware of the "on-off" phenomenon and increased involuntary abnormal movements, and told to notify his physician if they appear. The patient should also be aware that L-dopa darkens urine and sweat. Advise him to avoid pyridoxine (vitamin B_6), since it will increase peripheral conversion of L-dopa to dopamine.

The patient receiving amantadine should likewise be made aware of its action, dosage, and side effects. Caution him not to discontinue the drug abruptly, because that may worsen his parkinsonian symptoms. Since amantadine may cause insomnia, the last daily dose should not be taken near bedtime. Teach the patient how to deal with orthostatic hypotension.

With antihistamines and anticholinergic agents (Table 10-1), the patient should be cautioned to drive and operate machinery with care because these drugs cause drowsiness. Dry mouth can be alleviated with hard candy or chewing gum. These drugs should be given with or following meals. If he's receiving long-term therapy, the patient needs to be given frequent eye examinations, since this therapy is contraindicated with glaucoma.

C. Amyotrophic lateral sclerosis (ALS)

1. Description

Amyotrophic lateral sclerosis is a progressive neurologic disease that causes degenerative changes within the brain and spinal cord.

2. Etiology

The cause of ALS is unknown, although some theories suggest a link to either genetic defects, toxic metals, trauma, vitamin or enzyme deficiencies, an abnormal immune response, or a slow virus.

3. Incidence

The onset of ALS is usually between 50 and 70 years of age, with men affected two to three times more often than women. ALS affects approximately 1.4/100,000 population in the United States.

4. Pathophysiology

ALS produces degeneration of the cell bodies of the lower motor neurons of the spinal cord, and motor nuclei of cranial nerves in the brain stem. The cranial nerves most affected are V, VII, IX, X, XI, and XII, along with the lateral and ventral fiber tracts of the spinal cord. The corticospinal tract is the most severely affected. Degeneration of the cord is usually bilateral, though not symmetrical. The denervation that results from this disease causes atrophy of the muscles, but rarely affects the sensory pathways or mental faculties.

5. Signs and symptoms

Symptoms of ALS usually begin slowly and insidiously. The disease affects upper and lower motor neurons, with no specific degenerative patterns, so symptoms vary from person to person. The first indication may be irregular muscular twitchings (fasciculations) and muscle weakness, usually in the hands and feet. As the disease progresses, coordination is affected, and the muscles of the extremities become spastic and weak until flaccidity and atrophy occur.

With brain stem involvement, the muscles of the tongue, palate, pharynx, neck, and shoulders are impaired, making it difficult to chew, swallow, and speak. Paralysis eventually occurs in the affected muscles.

The patient may laugh or cry involuntarily, although mentation is intact. The senses of touch, sight, and hearing are not impaired.

In the terminal stages of the disease, weakened respiratory muscles cause shortness of breath and respiratory insufficiency. Death usually results from respiratory failure or bulbar paralysis.

6. Prognosis

Death usually occurs within 3 to 5 years. With early bulbar involvement, death can occur within 1 to 2½ years. Disability occurs sooner with bulbar involvement (several months) than with spinal cases (up to 4 years). Some ALS patients have survived for 10 to 15 years.

7. Diagnosis

Diagnosis is usually made from the history and neurologic examination. Other studies include electromyography, nerve conduction studies, creatine kinase level (elevated), and muscle biopsy. Other neurodiagnostic studies, such as myelogram, EEG, and brain scan, may be done to rule out other diseases.

8. Medical management of the patient with ALS

There is no treatment available to arrest or cure ALS, although individual symptoms are treated. Physical therapy may be ordered to minimize atrophy and development of contractures. Specialized appliances may be required.

Medications such as neostigmine (Prostigmin) or propantheline bromide (Pro-Banthine) may be given in small amounts to decrease bulbar weakness. Dantrolene or diazepam may be ordered for spasticity. If excessive salivation occurs, trihexyphenidyl (Artane) or amitriptyline (Elavil) may be administered.

Inability to swallow may require insertion of a nasogastric tube, cervical esophagostomy, or gastrostomy.

9. Nursing assessment of the patient with ALS

In the early stages of ALS, your goal is to support the patient and family and provide the education the family may need to care for the patient, with professional support, after discharge. In the terminal stage of the disease, support and comfort should be your primary goal. Following is a list of patient needs and suggestions for meeting them.

a. Communication. You'll need to assess the extent of the problem. A speech therapist is helpful. Take time and listen carefully as the patient speaks. Use letter or picture boards. An electrolarynx may be utilized in the earlier stages. Communication with hand squeezing or eye blinking may be necessary in the later stages. Provide the patient with a soft, pillow-like nursing call bell. Remember that the patient can hear and is completely aware of what is happening. The inability to communicate is frightening. Check on him often and reassure him that you will do this.

b. Nutrition. A dietitian and – again – a speech therapist can be helpful. A soft diet with six small daily meals may be ordered. Be sure the patient's fluid intake is adequate. High-protein supplements may be necessary. Have suction equipment available in case of choking, to prevent aspiration. Test the patient's ability to swallow before every meal. Allow plenty of time for him to eat. Teach the family how to feed the patient. If the patient is receiving his nutrition through a nasogastric tube, cervical esophagostomy, or gastrostomy, teach the family proper care of the tube and/or stoma if the patient will be returning home.

c. Respiratory needs. Evaluate the patient's respiratory status often. Encourage good posture. Elevate the head of the bed. Have the patient breathe deeply and cough frequently. Oxygen therapy may be necessary.

In the later stages of ALS, frequent suctioning is necessary to remove secretions. Prevent neck hyperextension. Fowler's or semi-Fowler's position is necessary at all times. Oxygen therapy will be administered.

d. Elimination. Determine the patient's normal bowel habits. You may prevent constipation by increasing fluid intake and including roughage in his diet. A stool softener may be ordered. Suppositories, laxatives, or enemas may occasionally be necessary, and the family should be taught to administer these.

e. Activity/immobility. Encourage activity for as long as possible, but also provide rest periods. Physical therapy is important. Active and passive exercises should be performed and taught to the family. A cane, walker, splints, or a wheelchair may be needed. Other aids, such as specialized feeding utensils, can be obtained with the help of an occupational therapist.

Evaluate the need for specialized equipment, such as railings and elevated toilet seats, in the home. Any articles in the home that will make mobility dangerous or difficult, such as scatter rugs, should be removed.

f. Comfort. The patient may experience pain from muscle spasms and cramps, and may need to have muscle relaxants and analgesics prescribed. Frequent skin care with massage can provide comfort as well as improve circulation and prevent skin breakdown. Turn the patient every 2 hours. Proper positioning with the use of a specialized mattress is necessary. Give mouth care frequently. Remember to teach the family these techniques to be continued at home.

g. Emotional needs. Depression is a frequent occurrence. Provide an atmosphere that will allow the patient and family to express their fears, concerns, and needs. Continued encouragement is necessary. Evaluate the patient's and family's ability to cope, and help provide psychiatric help should a problem arise. Be sure to provide the family with the teaching they require to help make the return home less stressful.

h. Discharge. Before the ALS patient returns home, a community health nurse should be contacted to assist the family. Be sure necessary equipment is arranged for. And let the family know what other services are available on an outpatient basis.

QUIZ

1. Which of the following does *not* describe the pathophysiology of multiple sclerosis?
   a. Degenerative changes in the cell bodies
   b. Initial breakdown of myelin
   c. Formation of scar tissue
   d. Degeneration of nerve fibers

2. Which of the following symptoms might a patient with MS have?
   a. Muscle spasticity
   b. Numbness
   c. Aphasia
   d. Loss of judgment
   e. Diplopia

3. The course of MS is characterized by _____ and _____.

4. Which of the following interventions might you include in your care plan for the patient with MS?
   a. Allow time for rest periods
   b. Help him accept the fact that his condition will progressively worsen
   c. Apply cold packs to spastic muscles
   d. Increase fluid intake

5. Parkinson's disease is a degenerative disease of the _____ that results in decreased production and storage of _____.

6. Symptoms of Parkinson's disease include:
   a. Muscle rigidity
   b. Muscle spasms
   c. Shuffling gait
   d. Intentional tremors

7. Treatment of Parkinson's disease with L-dopa can result in the following:
   a. Increased need for dietary protein
   b. Temporary worsening of symptoms with long-term use
   c. Development of jaundice
   d. Development of abnormal involuntary movements

8. The patient with Parkinson's disease may experience difficulty with:
   a. Mobility
   b. Communication
   c. Elimination
   d. Nutrition
   e. All of the above

9. Amyotrophic lateral sclerosis causes degeneration of the _____ cells in the spinal cord and brain stem.

10. Which of the following describe the signs and symptoms of ALS?
    a. Occur rapidly
    b. Vary from person to person
    c. Muscles become spastic and weak, then flaccid and atrophic
    d. Mentation is affected

11. In managing the patient with ALS, you should:
    a. Encourage deep breathing and coughing
    b. Check ability to swallow before meals
    c. Keep the patient on bed rest
    d. Evaluate the family's ability to care for the patient

ANSWERS
1. a.
2. a, b, d, e.
3. Remissions; exacerbations.
4. a, c, d.
5. Basal ganglia; dopamine.
6. a, c.
7. b, d.
8. e.
9. Motor.
10. b, c.
11. a, b, d.

CHAPTER

11

Neuromuscular Diseases

OBJECTIVES

After completing this chapter, you will be able to:

1. Discuss the pathophysiology and course of myasthenia gravis, as well as its signs and symptoms
2. Describe Guillain-Barré syndrome, including its pathophysiology, signs and symptoms, prognosis, and diagnostic measures
3. Discuss the course of carpal tunnel syndrome
4. Discuss nursing management goals for patients with myasthenia gravis, Guillain-Barré syndrome, and carpal tunnel syndrome.

A. Introduction

Although there is a large variety of diseases that affect nerves and muscles, we'll discuss here only the more significant, well-known problems.

B. Myasthenia gravis

1. Definition

Myasthenia gravis is a specific disease in which excessive weakness develops in involuntary muscles after repetitive stimulation or prolonged tension. Motor power is generally recovered after a period of inactivity or relaxation.

2. Incidence

Myasthenia gravis affects approximately three to six individuals per 100,000. It is most prevalent in women up to the age of 40. After 40, men and women are affected about equally. Although the disease is not hereditary, infants born to myasthenic mothers may exhibit temporary symptoms of the disease.

3. Pathophysiology and course

The basic mechanism in myasthenia gravis is a decrease of acetylcholine receptors on the postsynaptic membrane. This impairs transmission of nerve impulses, preventing normal muscle contraction.

The onset of myasthenia gravis is usually gradual. In some patients, it takes a mild course with little or no progression; in others, the course is rapid and difficult. Exacerbations and remissions are common.

4. Signs and symptoms

The chief symptom is progressive weakness, ranging from mild to severe, as muscles are used. Weakness generally is worse in the evening than in the morning. The first muscles to be affected are usually those of the eyes, and common symptoms are ptosis, diplopia, and ocular palsy. Next the muscles of the face and neck become involved. Chewing, swallowing, and speaking become difficult, and the head may need support. The trunk and limbs may follow, with proximal muscles affected more severely than distal muscles. Sitting and walking become difficult.

In severe myasthenia, abdominal and respiratory muscles become involved. Respiratory weakness may lead to death.

5. Classification

a. Group I: ocular myasthenia. This type involves only the ocular muscles, causing ptosis and diplopia. Patients have a high rate of remission, but respond poorly to medication.

b. Group IIA: mild myasthenia. Onset is slow, with no involvement of respiratory muscles. Patients respond well to medication and remissions are possible.

c. Group IIB: moderate myasthenia. Onset is slow, with more severe bulbar symptoms and skeletal muscle involvement. There is a poorer response to drugs, but remissions are still possible.

d. Group III: acute, severe myasthenia. There is a rapid onset of weakness in the skeletal and respiratory muscles. Myasthenic and cholinergic crises often occur, and the patient deteriorates rapidly. The mortality rate is high.

e. Group IV: late, severe myasthenia. In this type, severe symptoms develop within 2 years after one of the previous types of myasthenia. Deterioration can take place gradually or suddenly. There is a poor response to drugs and a high mortality rate.

6. Diagnosis

Myasthenia gravis is diagnosed by specific tests and by a history of muscle weakness.

a. Edrophonium (Tensilon) test. This test is useful if the weakness — like ptosis — can be easily observed. The test is performed by intravenous administration of edrophonium, a short-acting anticholinesterase drug. If the test is positive, muscle tone improves quickly, but for only about 5 minutes. Smaller doses of edrophonium are used for diagnosing cholinergic crises.

b. Neostigmine (Prostigmin) test. Neostigmine is a slowly acting anticholinesterase drug that produces its effects in about 30 minutes. It can be administered if the action of edrophonium is too short to produce or sustain increased muscle tone.

c. Electromyography (EMG). With EMG, 95 percent of myasthenic patients will show a characteristic pattern.

7. Nursing assessment of the patient with myasthenia gravis

Establish a baseline for ongoing assessment of muscle weakness by determining which muscles are affected, and whether they improve with rest.

Check for signs of diplopia and ptosis, and evaluate for any facial muscle weakness. Ask the patient whether he has problems chewing and swallowing and what he can eat without difficulty. Assess his ability to speak clearly.

Finally, determine the patient's tidal volume and vital capacity. Take note of the medications prescribed, their time schedule, and the presence of any side effects.

Because there is no cure for myasthenia gravis, management of the disease depends mainly on drug therapy — usually anticholinesterase drugs and, occasionally, corticosteroids. Other therapies include plasmapheresis and thymectomy.

a. Anticholinesterase drugs. These drugs inhibit the destruction of acetylcholine by cholinesterase, thereby increasing its accumulation at the myoneural junction. The most common anticholinesterase drugs are neostigmine and pyridostigmine (Mestinon).

As a result of their parasympathetic stimulant effect, these drugs have many side effects to be alert for (see Appendix).

b. Corticosteroids. The effectiveness of these drugs against myasthenia gravis may be secondary to their action on the immune system. Anticholinesterase drugs are given along with steroids.

Prednisone therapy usually consists of long-term, high-single-dose (100 mg), alternate-day administration. This dose is gradually tapered to the lowest amount that maintains normal function. Daily administration is sometimes tried.

ACTH increases circulating corticosteroid levels. It's usually given in an IV or IM dose of 100 units/day for 10 days and is generally reserved for patients who have not responded to oral steroids, anticholinesterase drugs, or thymectomy. Symptoms usually worsen during the first 3 days of therapy but then improve, even after therapy is completed. This drug-induced remission may last 3 to 6 months.

c. Other medications. Atropine counteracts the effects of anticholinesterase drugs and should be available for patients on them. For patients on steroids, potassium supplements and antacids are helpful in counteracting side effects.

d. Plasmapheresis. This procedure makes use of a specialized machine to remove the plasma from the patient's blood cells and return the cells to his body along with a plasma substitute. The principle is removal of circulating antibodies specific for acetylcholine receptors. It is effective in some patients — occasionally dramatically so.

e. Thymectomy. Thymoma is present in about 10 percent of myasthenia patients, and another 80 percent have thymic hyperplasia. It's thought that the thymus may initiate an autoimmune response to acetylcholine receptors. Thymectomy results in improvement in about 57 to 87 percent of patients, and produces remissions in 20 to 30 percent. Improvement may not, however, be clinically noticeable for 1 to 10 years.

8. Cholinergic crisis and myasthenic crisis

a. Cholinergic crisis. A cholinergic crisis is an acute reaction to overmedication with anticholinesterase drugs. Symptoms include diaphoresis, pupil constriction, salivation, nausea, vomiting, abdominal cramps, diarrhea, and bradycardia, in addition to severe muscle weakness. The patient may have acute respiratory distress, possibly leading to respiratory arrest and death. Immediate respiratory assistance is required.

b. Myasthenic crisis. Myasthenic crisis is characterized by severe motor weakness due to undermedication or lack of medication. This causes acute weakness of voluntary muscles and respiratory distress.

c. Diagnosis of crisis. The type of crisis—cholinergic or myasthenic—must be diagnosed in order to determine treatment. The edrophonium test is generally done. If injection of edrophonium makes the patient's condition worse, he's in cholinergic crisis. If he improves, he was in myasthenic crisis.

d. Treatment of crisis. Both types of crisis require respiratory assistance, depending on the extent of respiratory distress, as well as supportive measures to maintain body functions. Appropriate medications should be given as soon as the type of crisis is determined.

9. Nursing management of the patient with myasthenia gravis

Patients with this disease often need help with activities of daily living. Your goals are to promote adequate nutrition, help the patient manage ocular difficulties, administer drugs properly, maintain an airway, prevent gastrointestinal problems, and help the patient communicate. Emotional support and patient education are important aspects of your role. Chapter 5 discusses these measures in detail.

C. Guillain-Barré syndrome
1. Definition

Guillain-Barré syndrome—also known as Landry-Guillain-Barré-Strohl syndrome, infectious polyneuritis, or acute idiopathic polyneuritis—is a rare, reversible, paralytic disease of unknown etiology. It affects a variety of peripheral nerve roots and generally develops a few days to several weeks after a mild febrile illness. One hypothesis suggests that it is an autoimmune reaction.

2. Incidence

The incidence of this syndrome is 1.7/100,000. It occurs in persons of either sex and any age, but is most prevalent among young adults.

3. Pathophysiology

Edema of nerves, with degeneration of axons and myelin, can involve entire reflex arcs. Anterior and posterior nerve roots and peripheral and cranial nerves can be affected. Inflammatory reactions can be seen in the anterior horn cells and nuclei of cranial nerves.

4. Signs and symptoms

The clinical picture of Guillain-Barré syndrome varies from patient to patient. Symptoms can range from mild to severe.

Typically, the onset is abrupt. "Pins and needles" sensations in the hands and feet are followed by symmetrical muscle weakness and pain in the lower extremities. Flaccid ascending symmetrical paralysis develops within hours to days, accompanied by sensory loss in the extremities. Sensory disturbances include pain, paresthesias, and decrease in position and vibratory sense.

If the trunk becomes involved, urinary retention, constipation, and respiratory paralysis can result. Facial paralysis can occur with involvement of cranial nerve VII (facial). Involvement of cranial nerves IX (glossopharyngeal), X (vagus), XI (spinal accessory), and XII (hypoglossal) can cause difficulty in swallowing, talking, and chewing. If the vagus nerve is involved, the patient will experience unstable blood pressure with postural hypotension, facial flushing, extreme warmth, bradycardia, tachycardia, and diaphoresis.

Rarely do cerebral symptoms occur. Vision, hearing, eye movement, and sphincter control are not impaired.

5. Prognosis

The disease is self-limiting. About 95 percent of patients recover completely in a few weeks or months, although occasionally weakness in a limb or cranial nerve can continue. Motor function tends to return in a descending pattern. For some patients, recovery may be very slow, extending over a year or more. In the rare cases that are fatal, death usually results from respiratory failure or respiratory complications.

6. Diagnosis

A complete history, including previous illnesses, is important. A thorough physical exam should discover signs and symptoms previously described. A lumbar puncture is done to examine the cerebrospinal fluid. Initially the spinal fluid may be normal, but albuminocytologic dissociation — an increase in cerebrospinal fluid protein without an increase in white cell count — takes place within 4 to 6 weeks after onset.

7. Medical management of the patient with Guillain-Barré syndrome

There is no specific therapy for Guillain-Barré syndrome, although steroids may be given early in the disease to reduce edema and decrease the inflammatory response. Supportive measures include respiratory assistance with intubation (usually tracheostomy) performed when vital capacity drops to 25 to 30 percent of normal; use of antihypotensive drugs as needed; prophylactic anticoagulation with low-dose heparin or warfarin (Coumadin) to prevent thromboembolic complications of immobility; nutritional support through nasogastric feedings; and physical therapy.

8. Nursing assessment of the patient with Guillain-Barré syndrome

Because of the progressive nature of this syndrome, nursing assessment for changes in status is important. Assess respiratory function frequently; measure vital capacity, tidal volume, and forced inspiratory capacity every 4 hours. Evaluate the patient's level of consciousness, since it may be affected by hypoxia. Look for evidence of confusion, air hunger, and dyspnea. Assess neurologic function by evaluating the level of sensory and motor loss and the functioning of cranial nerves VII, IX, X, XI, and XII.

Monitor vital signs frequently, especially for alterations in blood pressure and pulse rate and rhythm. A cardiac monitor may be used to detect arrhythmias.

9. Nursing management of the patient with Guillain-Barré syndrome

The patient's clinical course and eventual recovery depend almost entirely on the effectiveness of nursing care. Because the course of this disease can vary greatly, nursing care is highly individualized. Your goals should center on observation for changes in status, maintenance of respiratory function, prevention of hazards of immobility, nutritional support, maintenance of musculoskeletal function, facilitating communication, and emotional support. Refer to Chapter 5 for specific interventions in these areas.

10. Rehabilitation

In the recovery phase, muscle strength begins to return, pain decreases, the autonomic nervous system stabilizes, and sensation returns. Rehabilitation measures center on improving muscle strength and on relearning activities of daily living.

D. Carpal tunnel syndrome

1. Description

Carpal tunnel syndrome is an entrapment syndrome due to irritation or compression of the median nerve within the carpal tunnel.

2. Pathophysiology

The carpal tunnel, located in the wrist, is formed by the carpal bones on three sides and on the other side by the transverse carpal ligament. The median nerve and blood vessels pass through the carpal tunnel. The median nerve innervates the muscles of thumb opposition, several hand muscles, and sensation in the first three digits. Any swelling of the contents of the carpal tunnel or change in its bony structure can affect the median nerve.

3. Signs and symptoms

Initially, compression of the median nerve causes sensory symptoms. The patient may complain of numbness, tingling, or burning of the hand and fingers, usually at night. The symptoms will then occur in the daytime and progress to loss of light touch sense and dulling to pinprick. Eventually, the motor component becomes involved, with clumsiness of the thumb and muscle wasting along the median nerve distribution. Pain becomes constant.

4. Etiology

The exact etiology of carpal tunnel syndrome is unknown. It is associated with conditions that can affect the size of the carpal tunnel or increase the volume of its contents. Hormones may play a role; some disorders associated with carpal tunnel syndrome include diabetes mellitus, rheumatoid arthritis, acromegaly, and myxedema. A history of wrist trauma is rare. Persons in certain occupations that require the wrist to move forcefully or to be placed in abnormal positions — for example, typists, hairdressers, and pianists — may be predisposed to the syndrome.

5. Incidence

Onset can occur at any age. There is an increased incidence in the sixth decade of life. The majority of those affected are women over 40.

6. Diagnosis

Diagnosis can be made on the history and on positive Phalen's and Tinel's signs. A positive Phalen's sign occurs when numbness and paresthesia begin or worsen along the median nerve after the wrists are held in flexion for a minute. To elicit Tinel's sign, tap the wrist lightly at the median nerve. A positive response is tingling radiating into the palm. Electromyography and nerve conduction studies are often done to rule out lesions of or near the spinal cord.

7. Management of the patient with carpal tunnel syndrome

Patients with carpal tunnel syndrome may be treated conservatively or may require surgery. Conservative treatment includes avoiding repetitive activities that utilize the wrist; utilizing a hand-wrist splint, primarily at night, to avoid wrist flexion; cortisone injections into the carpal tunnel for short-term relief; use of diuretics to reduce edema; and treatment of systemic disease if one is identified. If conservative therapy is begun, your role includes explaining activities to be avoided, use of the splint, and medications, if utilized.

Surgical decompression of the median nerve is indicated if conservative measures fail or if the condition worsens, causing damage to the motor component of the nerve. Following surgery, the paresthesia usually disappears but return of muscle strength and sensation may take several months. The amount of improvement and the length of time it takes depend on the amount of damage to the median nerve.

8. Nursing management of the patient with carpal tunnel syndrome

Before surgery, reinforce the surgeon's explanation of the procedure. Surgery may be done under general or local anesthesia. Postoperatively, the patient will return from the recovery room with a pressure dressing of gauze wrapped with an Ace bandage.

Follow the normal routine of checking postoperative vital signs. Elevate the affected hand with a pillow. Note the presence of sensation, movement, and circulation hourly in the affected fingers. Encourage the patient to exercise his fingers every hour by making a fist and relaxing it. The patient may experience moderate pain requiring an analgesic. The surgeon will order the Ace bandage removed several hours after surgery or the next day.

The patient is usually discharged the day after surgery. Discharge teaching is important. Tell the patient to avoid getting his dressing wet, and to keep the incision clean and dry. Instruct the patient to elevate his hand as much as possible; a sling is helpful for this purpose. Teach the patient how to check finger sensation and mobility as well as capillary refill of fingernails and how to slowly increase the activity of his affected hand after discharge. Usually the bandage and sutures are removed in 2 weeks and patients can return to work in 2 to 4 weeks.

QUIZ

1. The basic mechanism in myasthenia gravis is a decrease of _____ receptors on the _____ membrane.

2. Which of the following signs and symptoms can be found in a patient with myasthenia gravis?
   a. Inability to close eyelids
   b. Weakness of neck muscles
   c. Diplopia
   d. Paresthesias

3. Which of the following problems might you encounter in your care of the patient with myasthenia?
   a. Vision problems
   b. Cardiovascular difficulty
   c. Gastrointestinal problems
   d. Urinary retention

4. Which of the following are signs and symptoms of Guillain-Barré syndrome?
   a. Flaccid hemiplegia
   b. Loss of pain sensation
   c. Ascending paralysis
   d. Decrease in vibratory sense

5. Your nursing assessment of the patient with Guillain-Barré syndrome will include:
   a. Monitoring arterial blood gases
   b. Observing for signs of crisis
   c. Observing for cardiac arrhythmias
   d. Evaluating level of consciousness

6. Carpal tunnel syndrome is due to compression of the _____ nerve.

7. Following surgery for carpal tunnel syndrome, your care will include:
   a. Keeping the extremity elevated
   b. Immobilizing the affected hand and fingers
   c. Administering an analgesic
   d. Checking neurovascular status of the fingers

ANSWERS

1. Acetylcholine; postsynaptic.
2. **a, b, c.**
3. **a, c.**
4. **c, d.**
5. **a, c, d.**
6. Median.
7. **a, c, d.**

CHAPTER 12

Diagnostic Procedures

OBJECTIVES

After completing this chapter, you will be able to:

1. Identify the indications for a number of common neurologic diagnostic procedures

2. Discuss pretest nursing assessment

3. Describe certain neurologic diagnostic procedures

4. Perform post-test nursing assessment.

A. Introduction

Having obtained a detailed history and completed a thorough physical exam in order to begin to identify the patient's neurologic problems, the physician generally orders one or more diagnostic procedures to confirm and pinpoint the diagnosis. If noninvasive tests prove insufficient, invasive procedures may follow.

Many institutions require that patients sign consent forms before undergoing any invasive procedure. Be sure you're up to date on current hospital policy, to protect the patient, the institution, the physician — and yourself.

This chapter will discuss the nursing care necessary before and after certain common neurologic diagnostic procedures as well as their general indications and brief summaries of techniques. In every case, explain to the patient the purpose of the study and what will happen to him before, during, and after it. Your reassurance and support are necessary to help the patient cope with any anxiety.

B. Noninvasive procedures

1. Skull X-ray

a. Indications. This study is usually done to identify gross abnormalities. Skull films can determine the presence of a skull fracture, any unusual calcification or bone erosion, the position of the pineal body, and any abnormal vascularity.

b. Patient preparation. Explain to the patient that the procedure is similar to a chest X-ray and that radiation will be minimal. Have the patient transported to the X-ray department in a wheelchair or on a stretcher, depending on his ability to stand.

c. Procedure. Anteroposterior and lateral views are usually taken, with other angles included as necessary.

d. Postprocedure nursing care. None is necessary.

2. Spine X-ray

a. Indications. This test is most commonly done if the patient has experienced back trauma or has complained of pain or motor or sensory impairment. Spine films can visualize abnormal calcification or erosion, collapsed vertebrae, fractures, dislocations, spondylosis, and spurs. Before a myelogram, a spinal X-ray is taken to determine any mechanical problems.

b. Patient preparation. Prepare the patient as you would for skull X-ray.

c. Procedure. Anterior, posterior, and lateral views can be taken of the cervical, thoracic, lumbar, and sacral regions of the spine.

d. Postprocedure nursing care. None is necessary.

3. Electroencephalogram (EEG)

a. Indications. This study detects and localizes abnormal electrical activity in the brain. It is used to diagnose seizure disorders, trauma, inflammatory disease, and degenerative processes of the brain.

b. Patient preparation. Reassure the patient that the procedure is safe and that he will not receive an electric shock.

Be sure the patient's hair is clean, and free of hairpins and clips; remove any wig or other hairpiece. Because hypoglycemia can cause abnormalities on EEG readings, the patient should eat his normal diet but avoid caffeine-containing coffee, tea, and cola drinks.

If needle electrodes are to be used, explain that they create a sensation similar to that produced when a single hair is pulled out. For a sleep study, explain to the patient that he may be sedated after he arrives at the EEG suite.

Medications may be withheld for 24 to 48 hours before an EEG. If the physician hasn't ordered this, tell the EEG technician what drugs the patient is taking; some may affect study results.

c. Procedure. The patient is usually transported to the EEG suite for the test, although portable EEGs are sometimes brought to critically ill patients.

To begin, the patient lies down on a table or is seated in a comfortable chair while the technician applies approximately 19 electrodes. Disc electrodes are applied to the scalp with collodion; needle electrodes are inserted subcutaneously. With the patient's eyes closed, a recording of electrical impulses discharged by the brain cells is taken. The patient is then asked to hyperventilate for 4 to 5 minutes in order to raise the pH of the blood, which may trigger seizure activity in a susceptible individual.

Next, photic stimulation, in which a flickering light is placed before the patient's closed eyes, is used in an effort to accentuate abnormal brain activity.

Patients in whom seizure disorders are suspected are given a sedative and the EEG is taken during sleep — a state that can precipitate abnormal EEG activity.

If abnormal activity is suspected in the temporal lobe region, nasopharyngeal electrodes are inserted through the nostrils to the nasopharynx, near which the uncus of the temporal lobe lies.

d. Postprocedure nursing care. Remove dried collodion by brushing the hair, applying nail polish remover to it, and finally washing it. Because the sedated patient can be expected to sleep for several hours, put up side rails for safety. Resume pretest orders and observe seizure precautions with susceptible patients.

4. Computed tomography of the brain (CT or CAT scan)

This safe, reliable test has helped replace certain older, invasive studies, such as the pneumoencephalogram. A CT scan displays horizontal views of the brain in cross-section, providing a great deal of important information about the structure and status of the brain.

a. Indications. CT scans facilitate the diagnosis of cerebral infarcts, hydrocephalus, cerebral atrophy, hemorrhage, abscesses, and intracranial lesions, such as neoplasms.

b. Patient preparation. The patient should be on a clear liquid diet the day of the test. Tell him he'll receive the same amount of radiation as he would from a chest X-ray. Warn him that the machine will make a clicking sound during scanning. Sedation may be ordered if the patient seems unable to remain still during the scan. Be sure to remove all earrings, metal hairpins, or clips; dentures may remain.

If a contrast medium is to be used, find out whether the patient is allergic to X-ray contrast medium, shellfish, or iodine. If so, the physician may order steroids or antihistamines beforehand. Tell the patient he'll be given a temporary intravenous infusion and should expect a hot sensation (flush) when the contrast is injected.

c. Procedure. A narrow X-ray beam scans the head, 1 degree at a time, until a 180-degree area has been recorded. With the aid of a computer, photon absorption data are recorded for the various tissues. The tissue densities are assigned numbers called absorption coefficients, a digital printout of which displays the results of the scan. A horizontal cross-section of the head is also displayed on a television screen. Bone appears white; air, black; and soft tissue, shades of gray that vary in density. Any alteration of normal density indicates pathologic change. Four or five scans are usually taken of the head. The results are stored on a magnetic disc.

As the procedure begins, the patient lies flat on a movable table, with his head in the scanning unit. After each scan the table slowly moves, withdrawing the patient's head from the scanner to allow progressive views of the brain. To ensure accurate results, the patient must remain immobile for the full minute each scan takes. If further enhancement of tissues is indicated, a contrast medium is injected intravenously and another set of scans is taken. Without contrast, a CT scan takes 20 minutes; with contrast, 30 to 60 minutes.

d. Postprocedure nursing care. Patients who have had a CT scan without contrast medium require no special care. Following a CT scan with contrast, force fluids to facilitate excretion of the medium. Side effects of contrast include nausea and vomiting, chills, headache, dermal allergic reactions, and respiratory difficulty. Observe the patient for any changes in neurologic status, such as alteration in level of consciousness, orientation to time, place, and person, motor weakness, and loss of visual fields.

5. Echoencephalography

This procedure utilizes ultrasound to determine the displacement of midline structures.

a. Indications. Echoencephalography detects shifts of cerebral midline structures that can occur as a result of subdural hematoma, massive cerebral infarction, intracerebral hemorrhage, or cerebral neoplasms.

b. Patient preparation. Reassure the patient that the procedure is safe and that he will feel pressure and a rubbing sensation as the transducer is moved about.

c. Procedure. This study utilizes an ultrasound generator and receiver. Echoes from deep structures are displayed on an oscilloscope, from which Polaroid pictures are taken.

Placed either seated or supine, the patient must not move until the procedure is over. A water-soluble gel is applied to the skull at a point 4 to 5 cm vertically above the external auditory meatus of each ear. When a transducer is placed on each side of the head, at right angles to the skull, a series of spikes representing the head's diameter are displayed on the oscilloscope.

A single transducer is then placed in three positions on the skull: point A, above the auditory canal; point B, superior to point A; and point C, perpendicular and frontal to point B. Oscilloscope displays are obtained for each of these areas. The recording made from echoes within the brain then helps determine the positions of the midline structures. A shift in midline echoes of 2.5 mm or greater suggests the presence of a lesion.

d. Postprocedure nursing care. Remove the gel by washing the patient's hair. No special observations are necessary. Resume pretest orders and precautions.

6. Brain scan

This is a simple procedure that utilizes a radioactive isotope to visualize lesions in the brain.

a. Indications. Brain scans are used as screening studies to aid in the diagnosis of tumors, cerebrovascular disease, trauma, and inflammation.

b. Patient preparation. Reassure the patient that the procedure is safe and that he will not be subjected to any radiation hazard.

c. Procedure. A radiopharmaceutical is usually injected intravenously; oral and intra-arterial routes are occasionally used. It takes about 2 hours for the radioisotope to reach peak level in the brain. At that time, the patient is asked to sit or lie down for the scan, which takes about 20 to 30 minutes. The patient must remain as still as possible during the scan because any movement can affect its results.

d. Postprocedure nursing care. Radiation precautions are unnecessary. Resume pretest orders.

7. Noninvasive regional cerebral blood flow

This test measures cerebral blood flow by determining, over time, the concentration of inhaled xenon 133 (^{133}Xe) that is carried through the blood in the brain.

a. Indications. The study is used for the diagnosis and evaluation of cerebrovascular function. It also helps in understanding the pathophysiology of such problems as headache, dementia, seizure, coma, and metabolic disorders. In subarachnoid hemorrhage, the study can determine the presence and degree of vasospasm.

b. Patient preparation. No physical preparation is necessary.

c. Procedure. With the patient lying on a padded table, the technician places 16 probes on his scalp. The probes fit tightly, but are not uncomfortable. After a clip has been placed on the patient's nose, he is asked to breathe deeply through a mouthpiece or mask. He proceeds to inhale ^{133}Xe gas for about 1 minute, then air for 10 minutes more.

The inhaled radioactive gas travels through the cerebral vascular system, then returns to the lungs and is exhaled.

Skull probes pick up the radioactivity counts, which are read in turn by a computer that uses the information to calculate cerebral blood flow.

d. Postprocedure nursing care. There is no need for radiation precautions or special care. Resume pretest orders.

C. Invasive procedures
1. Lumbar puncture (spinal tap)

In this procedure, cerebrospinal fluid (CSF) is withdrawn from the subarachnoid space.

a. Indications. Analysis of the various components of CSF aids in the diagnosis of many neurologic disorders and can point to hemorrhage or infection of the central nervous system. It is also used to insert dye for certain diagnostic studies, such as myelograms, and to administer spinal anesthetics or medications.

b. Patient preparation. Tell the patient he'll experience coldness and wetness from the antiseptic; a brief sting, followed by localized numbness, from the anesthetic injection; and pressure when the needle is inserted.

Place the patient in lateral recumbent position, with the head flexed toward the chest, the knees flexed to the abdomen, and the back on the edge of the bed. This position allows for the widest space between the lumbar vertebrae. Encourage the patient to breathe slowly and deeply through his mouth to facilitate relaxation.

c. Procedure. A lumbar puncture takes from 10 to 30 minutes and is usually performed in the patient's room. The physician chooses the puncture area, dons gloves, cleanses the skin with antiseptic, drapes the area, and numbs it with local anesthetic, using a lumbar puncture set. The spinal needle is inserted between the spinous processes of L_{3-4} or L_{4-5} into the subarachnoid space, at which time the flow of CSF is evaluated.

Next, the doctor attaches a stopcock and manometer to the spinal needle, causing CSF to flow into the manometer.

TABLE 12-1

NORMAL VALUES OF CEREBROSPINAL FLUID

Pressure	60-180 mm H_2O
Red blood cells	None
White blood cells	0-5 cells/ml
Total protein	15-45 mg/100 ml
Glucose	50-75 mg/100 ml
Sodium	141 mEq/liter
Potassium	3.3 mEq/liter
Chloride	118-132 mEq/liter
Calcium	2.5 mEq/liter

Opening pressure is determined at the point where CSF stops rising and begins to fluctuate. Three specimens of CSF, about 1 ml each, are obtained, and their color noted; they're then sent to the laboratory for analysis. Table 12-1 outlines the normal values of cerebrospinal fluid. A final pressure reading is then taken and the needle is removed. The site is covered with a sterile Band-Aid.

d. Postprocedure nursing care. The patient must remain on his back for 4 to 24 hours. The head should be level with the rest of the body. Observe for changes in vital signs, level of consciousness, orientation to time, person, and place, and motor and sensory ability.

Encourage fluid intake. Administer analgesics for headache, which may last for 24 hours to a week. Encourage the patient to remain supine. Chart any post-test reactions.

2. Myelography

A myelogram is an X-ray of the spinal cord and vertebrae after injection of a water-soluble or oil-based contrast medium.

a. Indications. Myelograms permit visualization of the spinal cord and subarachnoid space for tumors, adhesions, abscesses, herniations or protrusions of intervertebral discs, and any mechanical constriction by a bony lesion.

b. Patient preparation. Warn the patient that he's likely to feel pain during insertion of the anesthetic and pressure during placement of the spinal needle. He may also experience discomfort from positioning during the procedure.

Be sure to ascertain whether the patient is allergic to shellfish, iodine, or the contrast medium. If so, antihistamines or steroids may be ordered before the test. The patient may receive a clear liquid diet or be forbidden anything by mouth prior to the study. Take and record baseline vital and neurologic signs, noting motor and sensory status in particular. The patient should void prior to the study. Premedication, if ordered, is a mild sedative.

Myelograms utilizing a water-soluble contrast medium require discontinuance 48 hours before the test of all drugs that lower seizure thresholds, including neuroleptic drugs, major tranquilizers, MAO inhibitors, psychostimulants, and phenothiazines.

c. Procedure. Spinal X-rays are taken prior to the study. Lumbar puncture is done under fluoroscopy with the patient either sitting, in the lateral decubitus position, or prone with a pillow under the abdomen. Small amounts of spinal fluid are taken and sent to the laboratory for analysis. The patient is then placed prone with the head of the X-ray tilt table elevated to 30 degrees.

Oil-based or water-soluble contrast medium is injected into the subarachnoid space. Because neither medium mixes with CSF, both can be manipulated into any area of the subarachnoid space by gravity. With water-soluble contrast, the spinal needle is removed immediately after injection. With oil-based contrast, on the other hand, the needle remains in place for the entire procedure.

Tilting the table causes the contrast medium to travel into the cervical, thoracic, and lumbar regions. Fluoroscopy follows. X-rays are taken of the areas to be examined.

Water-soluble contrast is absorbed from the CSF and excreted by the kidneys. To remove oil-based contrast, the table is tilted to allow the contrast to pool around the spinal needle. The medium is then withdrawn with a syringe.

d. Postprocedure nursing care. The type of contrast medium used determines what care is necessary.

After a myelogram taken with water-soluble contrast, the patient's head must be elevated 15 to 30 degrees for 8 hours. Limit activity during that time to prevent CSF turbulence. Maintain bed rest for 24 hours.

Check vital signs and neurologic status frequently for 24 hours. Maintain seizure precautions and observe the patient for seizure activity. Encourage fluid intake and diet as tolerated. No phenothiazines are to be taken for 48 hours.

Side effects of the contrast medium include nausea, vomiting, and possible urine retention. Administer analgesics for headache.

The patient who has received oil-based contrast medium must lie flat for 24 hours. Check vital signs and neurologic status frequently. Encourage oral fluids and resume the pretest diet. Be alert for urine retention. Observe for signs of chemical meningitis, including stiff neck and mild fever. Administer analgesics for headache.

3. Cerebral angiography

This study provides visualization of extracranial and intracranial blood vessels following the injection of a contrast medium.

a. Indications. Indications for cerebral angiography include suspected structural abnormalities, such as aneurysm, arteriovenous malformation, vessel thrombosis and stenosis, or abnormal vessel growth in the area of a brain tumor; suspected vessel displacement secondary to tumor growth, hydrocephalus, or hemorrhage; and cerebral blood flow alterations, such as abnormal vascular shunts, collateral flow patterns, and delays in circulation time.

b. Patient preparation. Determine the presence of allergy to drugs, contrast medium, shellfish, or iodine. A clear liquid diet is given the day of the study to maintain hydration. Shave the area where the medium is to be injected, usually the groin. Take baseline vital signs and assess neurologic function for comparison later. Evaluate distal pulses on the extremity to be used as a puncture site. For direct carotid or vertebral puncture, measure and record neck circumference. Ask the patient to remove any dentures, earrings, hairpins, and eyeglasses.

c. Procedure. The patient is placed supine on the X-ray table. Restraints are applied to prevent inadvertent movement, and an intravenous line is inserted. The puncture site is cleansed, draped, and anesthetized.

A needle is then inserted into the artery. If a distant artery, such as the femoral or brachial, is used, a radiopaque catheter is inserted and advanced retrograde under fluoroscopy into the vessels to be studied. Contrast medium is injected; films are taken as it progresses through the cerebral circulation. With contrast injection, the patient may feel some warmth in the face and neck and possibly some head pain. The patient's neurologic status and blood pressure are monitored throughout the procedure.

After the catheter or needle is removed, firm pressure is applied to the puncture site for 10 to 15 minutes. Finally, a dressing is applied to the site.

d. Complications. The complications that can occur with cerebral angiography include cerebral emboli, vasospasm, seizures, stroke, hematomas at the insertion site, distal emboli, cardiac arrhythmias, hypotension, syncope, bradycardia, and allergic reactions to the contrast medium.

e. Postprocedure nursing care. Keep the affected extremity immobilized in extension for 8 hours. Take vital signs often until the patient is stable. Assess neurologic status frequently. Observe for seizure activity. Observe the puncture site for bleeding or hematoma. Check the distal pulse, temperature, and color of the extremity used for puncture. If neck puncture was performed, measure neck circumference and check often for signs of hematoma formation. Ice may be applied to the puncture site.

Resume pretest diet and encourage fluid intake. Check urine output for 24 hours. Administer analgesic as needed.

4. Electromyography (EMG)

Electromyography examines the electrical activity of peripheral nerves and muscle.

a. Indications. An EMG can aid in the diagnosis of problems of the motor unit of peripheral nerves. This includes diseases of anterior horn cells, nerve roots, nerves, neuromuscular junctions, and muscle fibers.

b. Patient preparation. Tell the patient that he may feel pain when the needle electrode is inserted. In addition, he will hear audio amplification that sounds like firecrackers.

c. Procedure. The patient lies supine. A single needle is inserted into the muscle or muscles to be studied. Many muscles may be examined.

Muscle electrical activity is observed on insertion of the needle; immediately after insertion; with the muscle at rest; with minimal muscle contraction; and with maximal muscle contraction. The electrical activity is magnified by an amplifier and viewed on an oscilloscope screen with simultaneous audio amplification. A permanent recording of both signals is made.

d. Postprocedure nursing care. Administer a mild analgesic if the patient complains of aches in the muscles studied. Observe for hematoma at needle insertion sites, though this occurs only rarely.

5. Nerve conduction studies

Nerve conduction studies record the conduction speed of peripheral nerve fibers.

a. Indications. These studies are used to evaluate myelination of the fast-conducting myelinated fibers. Some diseases such as Guillain-Barré syndrome or Charcot-Marie-Tooth disease, slow nerve conduction velocities by causing demyelinating peripheral neuropathies.

b. Patient preparation. Reassure the patient that the procedure is safe but may cause him to feel intermittent tingling sensations similar to static electricity. These sensations may be uncomfortable. The patient must lie still.

c. Procedure. With the patient supine, the skin of the limb to be studied is cleansed with antiseptic and an abrasive such as sandpaper is used to decrease surface resistance. Surface electrodes are then taped to the skin and an electrical stimulus is applied. The speed of conduction, in meters per second, is determined.

d. Postprocedure nursing care. No special care is required.

QUIZ

Match each diagnostic procedure with its purpose.

1. Skull film _____
2. Spine film _____
3. Electroencephalography _____
4. CT scan _____
5. Echoencephalography _____
6. Brain scan _____
7. Noninvasive regional cerebral blood flow _____
8. Lumbar puncture _____
9. Myelography _____
10. Cerebral angiography _____
11. Electromyography _____
12. Nerve conduction study _____

a. Helps detect shifts of cerebral midline structures
b. Enables visualization of spinal cord
c. Helps detect abnormal electrical activity in the brain
d. Helps diagnose tumors, cerebrovascular disease, trauma, and inflammation via radioactive isotope
e. Helps diagnose CNS hemorrhage or infection
f. Helps diagnose gross skull abnormalities
g. Helps diagnose diseases that slow nerve conduction
h. Helps diagnose cerebral vessel abnormalities
i. Helps assess cerebrovascular function
j. Helps diagnose intracranial lesions
k. Helps diagnose diseases that affect the motor unit of peripheral nerves
l. Helps diagnose vertebral abnormalities

13. Which of the following may be included in preparing the patient for an electroencephalogram?
   a. Give clear liquid diet prior to study
   b. Withhold drugs
   c. Wash hair
   d. Explain that electrodes are not uncomfortable

14. Which of the following may be included in preparing the patient for cerebral angiography?
   a. Prep skin of appropriate area
   b. Give nothing by mouth prior to the study
   c. Measure neck circumference
   d. Check pedal pulses

15. Which of the following procedures utilize a contrast medium?
   a. CT scan
   b. Echoencephalogram
   c. Myelogram
   d. Brain scan

16. Two studies that require insertion of a spinal needle into the subarachnoid space are _____ and _____.

17. Following a myelogram utilizing water-soluble contrast, which actions may be included in your nursing care?
   a. Keep patient flat in bed for 24 hours
   b. Check vital signs and neurologic status frequently
   c. Administer medications for nausea
   d. Encourage fluid intake

18. Which of the following studies may cause discomfort, requiring an analgesic after the test?
   a. Cerebral blood flow study
   b. Cerebral angiography
   c. Electromyography
   d. Brain scan

ANSWERS
1. f.
2. l.
3. c.
4. j.
5. a.
6. d.
7. i.
8. e.
9. b.
10. h.
11. k.
12. g.
13. b, c.
14. a, c, d.
15. a, c.
16. Lumbar puncture; myelogram.
17. b, d.
18. b, c.

APPENDIX

DRUGS USED FOR NEUROLOGIC PROBLEMS

Drug	Indications
Adrenocorticotropin (ACTH)—adenohypophysial hormone	Severe myasthenia gravis, acute exacerbations of MS
Amantadine (Symmetrel)—antiparkinsonism, antiviral drug	Treatment of parkinsonism
Aminocaproic acid (Amicar)	Prevention of clot breakdown after cerebral aneurysm bleed
Atropine—anticholinergic	Treatment of muscle tremor and rigidity in Parkinson's disease. Treatment of cholinergic crisis in myasthenia gravis
Baclofen (Lioresal)—skeletal muscle relaxant	Treatment of spasticity due to multiple sclerosis or spinal cord injury
Bethanechol (Urecholine)—cholinomimetic	Treatment of acute, nonobstructive urinary retention in multiple sclerosis
Carbamazepine (Tegretol)—anticonvulsant)	Treatment of seizures, relief of trigeminal neuralgia and pain in multiple sclerosis
Carbidopa/levodopa (Sinemet)	Treatment of Parkinson's disease
Cimetidine (Tagamet)	Prevention of gastric irritation due to steroid therapy

Side effects	Nursing implications
Most common: sodium retention, potassium depletion, hypervolemia, hypertension, ketosis, lipolysis, immunosuppression, mood elevation, skin rash	Observe for sensitivity reactions Weigh patient and check for edema daily Observe for electrolyte imbalance, elevated blood sugar, infection
Irritability, anxiety, nausea, dizziness, ataxia, confusion, mild depression, constipation, urinary retention, skin rash, orthostatic hypotension, congestive heart failure	Observe for side effects and abrupt decrease in effectiveness Do not discontinue abruptly or administer near bedtime
Nausea, cramping, diarrhea, dizziness, tinnitus, malaise, pruritus, headache, hypotension, thrombosis	Assess for leg pain, chest pain, or other signs of thrombosis
Dry mouth, visual disturbances, constipation, urinary retention, impotence, mydriasis, bradycardia, tachycardia, drowsiness, weakness, insomnia	Administer oral preparations with food Monitor vital signs Warn patient about drowsiness
Drowsiness, insomnia, lightheadedness, headache, fatigue, weakness, confusion	Avoid use in epileptics; lowers seizure threshold Reduce dosage slowly to prevent hallucinations Avoid use with impaired renal function Evaluate blood sugar Warn patient not to operate machinery or take drug with alcohol
Sweating, flushing, headache, nausea, vomiting, hypotension, wheezing, dyspnea, atrial fibrillation	Administer on empty stomach Monitor fluid intake and output, blood pressure, respiratory status
Drowsiness, dizziness, ataxia, nausea, blurred vision, diplopia, confusion, rash, abnormal liver function, muscle ache, blood dyscrasias, urinary difficulties	Evaluate blood counts, liver function tests, urinalysis, BUN With epileptics, withdraw drug slowly Warn patients to avoid hazardous tasks at start of therapy
See levodopa Addition of carbidopa reduces many systemic side effects	Observe for development of abnormal involuntary movements
Headache, fatigue, diarrhea, dizziness, rash, confusion, muscle pain, bradycardia, arrhythmias	Observe for untoward effects Administer with meals Allow at least 1 hour between cimetidine and antacid

Drug	Indications
Dantrolene (Dantrium)—skeletal muscle relaxant	Treatment of spasticity in multiple sclerosis, cerebral palsy, paralysis
Dexamethasone (Decadron, Hexadrol)—adrenal corticosteroid	Treatment or prevention of cerebral edema
Diazepam (Valium)	Relief of spasticity due to upper motor neuron disorders Treatment of status epilepticus
Heparin sodium—anticoagulant	Prophylaxis against thrombosis in immobile patients, and of cerebral thrombi in stroke-in-evolution
Levodopa (L-dopa, Larodopa)—antiparkinsonism drug	Treatment of Parkinson's disease
Mannitol (Osmitrol)—osmotic diuretic	Treatment of cerebral edema and increased intracranial pressure
Neostigmine (Prostigmin)—anticholinesterase	Diagnosis and treatment of myasthenia gravis
Prednisone—adrenal corticosteroid	Treatment of multiple sclerosis and myasthenia gravis
Pyridostigmine (Mestinon)—anticholinesterase	Treatment of myasthenia gravis
Urea (Ureaphil)—osmotic diuretic	Treatment of increased intracranial pressure
Vasopressin (Pitressin)—synthetic antidiuretic hormone	Treatment of diabetes insipidus

Side effects	Nursing Implications
Drowsiness, dizziness, weakness, fatigue, diarrhea, abdominal cramps, GI bleeding, hepatotoxicity, tachycardia	Observe for untoward effects Monitor liver function Warn patient to avoid hazardous tasks
See prednisone	See prednisone
Drowsiness, ataxia, lethargy, headache, vertigo, rash, nausea, urinary retention, bradycardia, tachycardia, blurred vision, edema, changes in libido	Withdraw drug slowly after long-term use Assess for excessive drowsiness Warn patient to avoid hazardous tasks and alcohol use Observe for signs of dependence
Hemorrhage, hypersensitivity, alopecia, osteoporosis, renal impairment	Rotate injection sites Monitor clotting time or partial thromboplastin time Observe for abnormal bleeding Check for blood in urine and stool
Nausea, vomiting, anorexia, orthostatic hypotension, palpitations, weakness, fatigue, hand tremor, insomnia, headache, confusion, anxiety, delusions, hallucinations, euphoria, "on-off" phenomenon, abnormal involuntary movements	Monitor renal, hepatic, cardiovascular function Assess blood sugar in diabetics Give drug with food Measure blood pressure supine and standing Warn patient to rise slowly Observe for abnormal involuntary movements and "on-off" signs
Dry mouth, thirst, headache, electrolyte imbalance, dehydration, hypotension, circulatory overload	Monitor urine output hourly Monitor electrolytes Avoid extravasation of solution; observe IV site for inflammation and edema Discard crystallized solution
Nausea, diarrhea, cramps, sweating and salivation, urinary urgency, muscle twitching, blurred vision, bradycardia	Observe for untoward reactions Give before meals or periods of increased activity Observe for cholinergic crisis
Salt and water retention, sweating, increased appetite, hypertension, gastrointestinal disturbances, rash, osteoporosis, mood changes, headache, vertigo	Observe for side effects Administer with food or milk Evaluate blood sugar and electrolytes often Observe for signs of infection Check stool for blood Withdraw drug gradually
See neostigmine	See neostigmine
Headache, nausea, syncope, confusion, electrolyte imbalance, tachycardia, hypotension	Monitor urine output hourly Avoid extravasation of solution
Pallor, nausea, gastrointestinal disturbances, uterine cramping, vertigo, sweating, headache, hypersensitivity, bronchoconstriction, angina	Observe for water intoxication (drowsiness, listlessness, headache, confusion) Monitor urinary specific gravity Monitor vital signs, daily weight, fluid intake and output

GLOSSARY

Abulia – inability to perform voluntary acts or make decisions

Agnosia – inability to recognize objects and symbols by means of the senses, although primary sensory receptors are intact

Anesthesia – complete loss of sensation

Anosmia – loss of sense of smell

Aphasia – loss or impairment of the ability to recognize, manipulate, or express words as symbols of ideas

Apraxia – loss of ability to perform purposeful movement, although comprehension is intact and motor and sensory dysfunction is absent

Astereognosis – inability to recognize an object by touch

Ataxia – inability to perform coordinated movements

Aura – a sensory phenomenon that may precede a convulsion

Bifurcation – division into two branches

Bulbar – pertaining to the medulla

Chorea – involuntary, irregular jerking movements

Clonic – spasmodic alternation of contraction and relaxation

Coma – a state of profound unconsciousness from which the patient cannot be aroused

Conjugate – working in unison

Contralateral – on the opposite side

Contrecoup – injury to the brain produced on the side opposite the original impact

Contusion – a bruise caused by a blow with a blunt object

Coup – injury to the brain produced on the side of the original impact

Craniotomy – an operation on the skull consisting of the removal and replacement of bone

Cranium – the skull

Decussate – to cross over

Delirium – behavior characterized by delusions, restlessness, disorientation, and incoherent speech

Dermatome – the area of skin supplied with afferent nerve fibers by a single posterior spinal root

Diplopia – double vision

Dysarthria – impairment of articulation by a disorder affecting the muscles of speech

Dysphagia – difficulty in swallowing

Dysphasia – impaired comprehension or expression of ideas (see Aphasia)

Fasciculations – spontaneous contractions of a number of muscle fibers supplied by a single motor nerve

Fissure – a deep fold

Flaccid – without tone; limp

Fusion – surgical union of bone with bone

Gyrus – elevations (convolutions) on the surface of the brain

Hemianopsia – loss of vision in one half of the visual field

Hemiparesis – muscular weakness affecting one side of the body

Hemiplegia – loss of motor ability on one side of the body

Homonymous hemianopsia – loss of vision in some portion of visual field for both eyes

Hydrocephalus – abnormal accumulation of cerebrospinal fluid within the cranium

Hypercapnia – excess of carbon dioxide in the blood

Ipsilateral – on the same side

Lamina – thin, dorsal part of the vertebra

Laminectomy – removal of the dorsal arches of the vertebrae to permit surgery on the spinal cord

Miosis – excessive contraction of the pupil

Nuchal rigidity – stiff neck

Nystagmus – involuntary, rapid movement of the eyes

Otorrhea – drainage of cerebrospinal fluid from the ear

Papilledema – swelling of the optic nerve head

Paralysis – loss of the ability of muscle to contract

Paraplegia – paralysis of the lower extremities

Paresis – slight or incomplete paralysis

Paresthesia – abnormal sensation (burning, itching, prickling, or crawling)

Ptosis – drooping of the upper eyelid

Quadriplegia – paralysis of all four extremities

Rhinorrhea – drainage of cerebrospinal fluid from the nose

Scotoma – a blind or partially blind area in the visual field

Spasticity – abnormal increase in muscle tone

Tentorium – a double fold of dura mater between the occipital lobes and the cerebellum

Tinnitus – ringing in the ears

Xanthochromia – yellow discoloration of cerebrospinal fluid due to disintegrated red blood cells

ADDITIONAL TEST QUESTIONS

1. If the electrical charges across the cell membrane are negative on the outside and positive on the inside, the cell is said to be:
   a. Saltatory
   b. Polarized
   c. Depolarized
   d. Refractory

2. A lesion in the precentral gyrus of the frontal lobe could result in which of the following symptoms?
   a. Motor paralysis
   b. Aphasia
   c. Blindness
   d. Deafness

3. Which of the following arteries is *not* part of the circle of Willis?
   a. Anterior communicating artery
   b. Middle cerebral artery
   c. Posterior cerebral artery
   d. Posterior communicating artery

4. Which cranial nerve is affected if the patient's pupils do not constrict when exposed to light?
   a. Optic
   b. Trochlear
   c. Oculomotor
   d. Abducens

5. Which of the following reactions does *not* occur with parasympathetic stimulation?
   a. Pupillary constriction
   b. Decrease in blood pressure
   c. Coronary artery constriction
   d. Increased heart rate

6. To evaluate abstract reasoning ability, you would ask the patient:
   a. The meaning of a proverb
   b. To repeat a number series
   c. To solve a problem of daily life
   d. To perform a simple act

7. While testing a patient's visual fields, which of the following would you *not* do?
   a. Sit 2 to 3 feet from the patient
   b. Dim the lights
   c. Ask the patient to cover one eye
   d. Direct him to look at your nose

8. To test the function of cranial nerve V, you would:
   a. Shine a light into the patient's pupils
   b. Ask the patient to smile, frown, whistle, blow out his cheeks
   c. Ask the patient to follow your fingers with his eyes
   d. Touch the patient on his face with a wisp of cotton

9. To test for cerebellar function, you would ask the patient to:
   a. Turn his chin against the resistance of your hand
   b. Walk heel to toe
   c. Identify familiar objects placed in his hand
   d. Identify numbers drawn on his palm

10. While evaluating a patient's gait, you notice that the left leg moves stiffly and outward in a semicircle. What disease process could cause this type of gait?
   a. Multiple sclerosis
   b. Parkinson's disease
   c. Stroke
   d. Cerebral palsy

11. Which of the following is an abnormal response during reflex testing?
   a. Ankle clonus when the foot is dorsiflexed
   b. Plantar flexion when the sole of the foot is stroked
   c. Elbow extension when the triceps tendon is tapped
   d. Knee extension when the patellar tendon is tapped

12. Which situation is considered a medical emergency?
   a. An increase in a Glasgow coma scale score from 9 to 15
   b. Absence of the corneal reflex in a patient in deep coma
   c. A change from decerebrate posturing to decorticate posturing
   d. A change from normally reacting pupils to a unilaterally dilated and unreactive pupil

13. Which of the following actions are *not* a part of the nursing management of the comatose patient?
   a. Position the patient in a chair for several hours
   b. Removal of splints every 4 hours
   c. Turning the patient every 2 hours from side to back to side
   d. Initiation of seizure precautions

14. Which symptom of increased intracranial pressure occurs least often?
   a. Vomiting
   b. Pupillary constriction
   c. Papilledema
   d. Hypertension

15. Which of the following factors can cause an increase in intracranial pressure?
   a. Hypocapnia
   b. Isometric exercises
   c. Passive range of motion exercises
   d. Deep breathing

16. While you were caring for Mr. Peters, he experienced a seizure. At first he complained of a buzzing sound followed by twitching of his right arm, which then spread throughout his body. Afterward, he was unconscious for a short period of time. What type of seizure did he experience?
   a. Complex partial seizure
   b. Generalized major motor seizure
   c. Myoclonic seizure
   d. Secondary generalized partial seizure

17. You suspect that your patient is experiencing anticonvulsant drug toxicity. Your neurologic assessment should specifically include evaluation of:
   a. Coordination
   b. Pupillary responses
   c. Sensory function
   d. Reflexes

18. During a tonic-clonic seizure, you should never:
   a. Elevate the patient's head
   b. Turn the patient
   c. Restrain the patient's movements
   d. Insert a padded tongue blade between his teeth

19. In your teaching of the epileptic patient, which of the following would you *not* tell him to do?
   a. Completely avoid alcohol
   b. Decrease his physical activity
   c. Never stop his medications
   d. Avoid fatigue

20. Which is the major problem that can occur as a result of status epilepticus?
   a. Aspiration
   b. Trauma
   c. Cerebral edema
   d. Cerebral anoxia

21. Which of the following actions should you avoid when feeding a patient with dysphagia?
   a. Feed the patient in the upright position with torso forward and head flexed
   b. Give plenty of fluids since they are easiest to swallow
   c. Avoid feeding milk products
   d. Include semisolids in the diet

22. A patient was brought into the emergency department with a diagnosis of possible stroke. Your first action would be to:
   a. Establish a patent airway
   b. Check vital signs
   c. Evaluate his neurologic status
   d. Obtain information from the family member who accompanied him

23. With cerebral aneurysm, the primary complication after the initial bleed is:
   a. Cerebral edema
   b. Seizures
   c. Rebleeding
   d. Vasodilation

24. Which of the following should you avoid when a patient has had a cerebral aneurysm bleed?
   a. Limit television and radio
   b. Take temperatures rectally
   c. Allow the patient to help with his bath
   d. Limit visitors

25. Mr. Thompson was admitted to your unit following bleeding from an anteriovenous malformation. Your nursing efforts will be focused primarily on prevention of:
   a. Seizure activity
   b. Hazards of immobility
   c. Headache
   d. Rebleeding

26. Ms. Hunter was admitted to the hospital following an auto accident. She was unconscious with a blood pressure of 200/100 and a pulse rate of 55. With no other information, you might suspect:
   a. Increased intracranial pressure
   b. Hemorrhagic shock
   c. Neurogenic shock
   d. Cervical injury

27. The purpose of hyperventilating a patient with increased intracranial pressure is to:
   a. Increase oxygen levels in the blood, thereby increasing oxygen supply to ischemic tissues
   b. Decrease carbon dioxide levels in the blood, which leads to constriction of cerebral arteries
   c. Increase oxygen levels in the blood, which leads to dilation of cerebral arteries
   d. Decrease carbon dioxide blood levels, which leads to cerebral artery vasodilation

28. One of the complications following head trauma is diabetes insipidus. What would you assess to determine whether this problem exists?
   a. Check blood sugar level
   b. Check urine for increased specific gravity and decreased amount
   c. Check urine for decreased specific gravity and increased amount
   d. Check urine for an increase in electrolytes

29. Ms. Roberts suffered a complete spinal cord injury at the T_2-T_4 level. Functionally, you would *not* expect her to:
   a. Perform self-catheterization
   b. Walk with long-leg braces
   c. Utilize a nonelectric wheelchair
   d. Become completely independent

30. As you participate in Ms. Roberts' rehabilitation, which of the following would you *not* encourage her to do?
   a. Increase fluids to 3000 ml/day
   b. Use stool softeners
   c. Hope to walk eventually
   d. Check her skin for pressure areas

31. Following a craniotomy, your patient developed bloody drainage from the ear. What would you do?
   a. Pack the ear with gauze
   b. Check the drainage for CSF with a Dextrostix
   c. Call the doctor immediately
   d. Check for CSF by observing for a clear ring around the blood on a towel

32. One of the primary symptoms of pituitary tumors is:
   a. Visual field defects
   b. Papilledema
   c. Hyperpituitarism
   d. Facial asymmetry

33. Which of the following symptoms would you *not* expect to result from chemotherapy for brain tumors?
   a. Bruising
   b. Constipation
   c. Mouth irritation
   d. Nausea

34. Which of the following statements regarding spinal cord tumors is *not* true?
   a. Cause cord compression rather than invasion
   b. Affect males and females equally
   c. Majority are malignant
   d. Rarely occur before age 10

35. In caring for a patient with a spinal cord tumor, your principal nursing goal would be:
   a. Relief of pain
   b. Prevention of deformities
   c. Prevention of respiratory difficulties
   d. Maintenance of skin integrity

36. Which of the following statements regarding multiple sclerosis is true?
   a. The disease progresses relentlessly to severe disability
   b. Exacerbations are predictable
   c. Stress can trigger an exacerbation
   d. It is caused by a virus

37. Your nursing care of the patient with MS should not include:
   a. Hot baths to decrease spasticity
   b. Active exercises
   c. Increasing fluid intake
   d. Intermittent catheterization

38. Parkinson's disease is due to:
   a. A decrease of dopamine in the presynaptic terminal
   b. An increase in reuptake of dopamine
   c. An increase in dopamine in the basal ganglia
   d. A decrease in production and storage of dopamine in the basal ganglia

39. Carbidopa is given with L-dopa to:
   a. Prevent conversion of L-dopa to dopamine in the basal ganglia
   b. Prevent conversion of L-dopa to dopamine in peripheral tissues
   c. Facilitate conversion of L-dopa to dopamine in the basal ganglia
   d. Facilitate conversion of L-dopa to dopamine in the peripheral tissues

40. Ms. Jackson, a patient with parkinsonism, stopped responding to L-dopa and her symptoms worsened. What alteration in her drug therapy might improve the situation?
   a. Increase her dosage of L-dopa
   b. Stop L-dopa for a short period
   c. Spread out the dosage of L-dopa
   d. Switch to another drug

41. The cause of death in patients with amyotrophic lateral sclerosis is usually:
   a. Transtentorial herniation
   b. Infection
   c. Cardiac failure
   d. Respiratory paralysis

42. ALS will *not* cause an impairment of the patient's ability to:
   a. Swallow
   b. Speak
   c. Hear
   d. Walk

43. Mr. Smith, a myasthenic patient, began to suffer increased muscle weakness and respiratory distress. His condition improved following administration of edrophonium. This problem may have occurred as a result of:
   a. Overmedication with prednisone
   b. Overdose of anticholinesterase drugs
   c. Undermedication with anticholinesterase drugs
   d. Undermedication with prednisone

44. When teaching the myasthenic patient about his medications, it is important to explain that he:
   a. Must *always* take them on time
   b. Should take them after meals
   c. Can occasionally miss a dose
   d. Will not need them for the rest of his life

45. Which of the following is not a symptom of Guillain-Barré syndrome?
   a. Flaccid symmetrical paralysis
   b. Pain
   c. Urinary retention
   d. Hemianopsia

46. Following surgery for carpal tunnel syndrome, the patient should be told *not* to:
   a. Exercise his fingers
   b. Elevate his hand
   c. Get his dressing wet
   d. Eat for 24 hours

47. You are preparing a patient for a myelogram. Which of the following would you *not* do?
   a. Shave the site
   b. Check allergy history
   c. Order a clear liquid diet
   d. Do a neuro check

48. Following a cerebral arteriogram, you would *not:*
   a. Apply ice to the puncture site
   b. Flex the affected extremity
   c. Encourage fluid intake
   d. Observe for seizure activity

49. Ms. C, who is unconscious, requires meticulous skin and hygienic care. Which of the following would you not include in your care plan?
   a. Toothbrushing
   b. Use of turning sheet
   c. Use of incontinence pads
   d. Turning every hour

50. Which of the following would not be part of your care plan after a lumbar puncture?
  a. Observing for neurologic change
  b. Encouraging fluid intake
  c. Administering analgesics
  d. Elevating the patient's head

ANSWERS

1. c.	26. a.
2. a.	27. b.
3. b.	28. c.
4. c.	29. b.
5. d.	30. c.
6. a.	31. d.
7. b.	32. a.
8. d.	33. b.
9. b.	34. c.
10. c.	35. a.
11. a.	36. c.
12. d.	37. a.
13. c.	38. d.
14. a.	39. b.
15. b.	40. b.
16. d.	41. d.
17. a.	42. c.
18. c.	43. c.
19. b.	44. a.
20. d.	45. d.
21. b.	46. c.
22. a.	47. a.
23. c.	48. b.
24. c.	49. c.
25. d.	50. d.

SELECTED READINGS

General references

Adams R, Victor M: *Principles of Neurology*, 2nd ed. New York: McGraw-Hill, 1981

Conway-Rutkowski BL: *Carini and Owens' Neurological and Neurosurgical Nursing*. St Louis: Mosby, 1982

Hickey JV: *The Clinical Practice of Neurological and Neurosurgical Nursing*. Philadelphia: Lippincott, 1981

Taylor J, Ballenger S: *Neurological Dysfunctions and Nursing Intervention*. New York: McGraw-Hill, 1980

Wehrmaker S, Wintermute J: *Case Studies in Neurologic Nursing*. Boston: Little, Brown, 1978

Chapter 1

Chusid J: *Correlative Neuroanatomy and Functional Neurology*, 17th ed. Los Altos, Ca: Lange Medical Publications, 1979

Clark RG: *Manter & Gatz's Essentials of Clinical Neuroanatomy and Neurophysiology*. Philadelphia: Davis, 1975

Guyton AC: *Textbook of Medical Physiology*, 5th ed. Philadelphia: Saunders, 1976

Noback C, Demarest R: *The Nervous System — Introduction and Review*. New York: McGraw-Hill, 1977

Chapter 2

Alpers B, Mancall E: *Essentials of the Neurological Examination*. Philadelphia: Davis, 1971

Bates B: *A Guide to Physical Examination*, 2nd ed. Philadelphia: Lippincott, 1979

Engel GL, Morgan WL Jr: *Interviewing the Patient*. Philadelphia: Saunders, 1973

Mitchell P, Irvin N: Neurological examination: Nursing assessment for nursing purposes. *J Neurosurg Nurs* 9:23, 1977

Chapter 3

Essentials of the Neurological Examination. Philadelphia: SmithKline Corp, 1974

Mechner F, et al: Programmed instruction. Patient assessment: Neurologic examination, part I. *Am J Nurs* 75:P.I.1, 1975

Mechner F, et al: Programmed instruction. Patient assessment: Neurologic examination, part II. *Am J Nurs* 75:P.I.1, 1975

Mechner F, et al: Programmed instruction. Patient assessment: Neurologic examination, part III. *Am J Nurs* 76:P.I.1, 1976

Chapter 4

Adams N: Prolonged coma: Your care makes all the difference. *Nursing*, p 21, Aug 1977

Allen N: Prognostic indicators in coma. *Heart Lung* 8:1075, 1979

Erickson R: Cranial check: A basic neurological assessment. *Nursing*, p 87, Aug 1974

Jimm L: Nursing assessment of patients for increased intracranial pressure. *J Neurosurg Nurs* 6:27, 1974

Jones C: Monitoring recovery after head injury: Translating research into practice. *J Neurosurg Nurs* 11:192, 1979

Loen M, Snyder M: Psycho-social aspects of care of the long-term comatose patient. *J Neurosurg Nurs* 11:235, 1979

Parsons L: Respiratory changes in head injury. *Am J Nurs* 71:2187, 1971

Plum F, Posner J, eds: *The Diagnosis of Stupor and Coma*, 3rd ed. Philadelphia: Davis, 1980

Snyder J, Powner D: Considerations in the medical care of neurologically impaired patients. *Heart Lung* 8:1065, 1979

Spielman G: Coma: A clinical review. *Heart Lung* 10:700, 1981

Chapter 6

Clark A: Antiepileptic drug update. *RN* 43:56, May 1980

Gastaut H: Clinical and electroencephalographical classification of epileptic seizures. *Epilepsia* 11:102, 1970

Hawken M: Seizures: Etiology, classification, intervention. *J Neurosurg Nurs* 11:166, 1979

Hawken M, Ozuna J: Practical aspects of anticonvulsant therapy. *Am J Nurs* 79:1062, 1979

Norman S: Surgical treatment of epilepsy. *Am J Nurs* 81:995, May 1981

Norman S, Brown T: Seizure disorders. *Am J Nurs* 81:984, May 1981

Swift N: Helping patients live with seizures. *Nursing* 8:24, June 1978

Tucker, CA: Complex partial seizures. *Am J Nurs* 81:996, 1981

Chapter 7

Allwood A, Lundy C: Cerebral artery bypass surgery. *Am J Nurs* 80:1284, 1980

Doolittle N: Arteriovenous malformations: The physiology, symptomatology, and nursing care. *J Neurosurg Nurs* 11:221, 1979

Gary R: Cerebral vasospasm: Process, trends and interventions. *J Neurosurg Nurs* 13:256, 1981

Hasgrove R: Feeding the severely dysphagic patient. *J Neurosurg Nurs* 12:102, 1980

Lee K: Aneurysm precautions: A physiologic basis for minimizing rebleeding. *Heart Lung* 9:336, 1980.

Norman S, Baratz R: Understanding aphasia. *Am J Nurs* 79:2135, 1979

Polhopek M: Stroke: An update on vascular disease. *J Neurosurg Nurs* 12:81, 1980

Sawitzke S, Teter A: Arteriovenous malformations of the brain. General review including role of embolization. *J Neurosurg Nurs* 8:132, 1976

Stillman M: Stroke! Pulling your patients through the acute phase. *RN* 42:55, Oct 1979

Chapter 8

Bailey J: Head trauma. *RN* 42:44, May 1979

Bowers S, Marshall L: Severe head injury: Current treatment and research. *J Neurosurg Nurs* 14:210, 1982

Carol M: Acute care of spinal cord injury: A challenge to the emergency medicine clinician. *Crit Care Q* 2:7, June 1979

Connolly R, Zewe G: Update: head injuries. *J Neurosurg Nurs* 13:195, 1981

Egan J: Rehabilitation: The nurse's responsibility in the intensive care unit. *Crit Care Q* 2:105, June 1979

King R, Dudas S: Rehabilitation of the patient with a spinal cord injury. *Nurs Clin North Am* 15:225, 1980

Kunkel J, Wiley J: Acute head injury: What to do when and why. *Nursing* 9:23, March 1979

Larrabee J: The person with a spinal cord injury: Physical care during early recovery. *Am J Nurs* 77:1320, 1977

Pepper G: The person with a spinal cord injury: Psychological care. *Am J Nurs* 77:1330, 1977

Stauffer S: A master-plan for teaching the patient with spinal cord injury. *RN* 42:55, July 1979

Tyson G, et al: Acute care of the head-injured patient. *Crit Care Q* 2:23, June 1979

Tyson G, et al: Acute care of the spinal-cord injured patient. *Crit Care Q* 2:45, June 1979

Chapter 9

Arsenault L: Primary spinal cord tumors: A review and case presentation of a patient with an intramedullary spinal cord neoplasm. *J Neurosurg Nurs* 13:53, 1981

Gehrke M: Identifying brain tumors. *J Neurosurg Nurs* 12:203, 1980

Larson E: The epidemiology of primary brain tumors. *J Neurosurg Nurs* 12:121, 1980

McQuat F: The insidious spinal cord tumor. *J Neurosurg Nurs* 13:18, 1981

Smith J, Geist B: Evaluation and care of the acute craniotomy patient. *J Neurosurg Nurs* 10:102, 1978

Stewart C: Current concepts of chemotherapy for brain tumors. *J Neurosurg Nurs* 12:97, 1980

Stillman M: Transphenoidal hypophysectomy for pituitary tumors. *J Neurosurg Nurs* 13:117, 1981

Tortorelli B: Acoustic neuroma: An overview of the disorder and nursing care for these patients. *J Neurosurg Nurs* 13:170, 1981

Wheeler P: Care of the patient with a cerebellar tumor. *Am J Nurs* 77:263, 1977

Chapter 10

Appel S: Multiple sclerosis – New ideas and a new test. *Heart Lung* 10:710, 1981

Blount M, et al: Management of the patient with amyotrophic lateral sclerosis. *Nurs Clin North Am* 14:157, 1979

Catanzaro M: Multiple sclerosis: Exploding myths that compromise patient care. *RN* 40:42, Dec 1977

Dolan B: Multiple sclerosis. *J Neurosurg Nurs* 11:83, 1979

Garrett E: Parkinsonism: Forgotten considerations in medical treatment and nursing care. *J Neurosurg Nurs* 14:13, 1982

Hartley F: A nurse's view: Amyotrophic lateral sclerosis. *J Neurosurg Nurs* 13:89, 1981

Holland N, et al: Overview of multiple sclerosis and nursing care of the M.S. patient. *J Neurosurg Nurs* 13:28, 1981

Kelly-Hayes M: Guidelines for rehabilitation of multiple sclerosis patients. *Nurs Clin North Am* 15:245, 1980

Lewis S, Lewis V: Multiple sclerosis: Does the mystery remain? *J Neurosurg Nurs* 11:176, 1979

Olsen B: Motor neuron disease: Amyotrophic lateral sclerosis. *J Neurosurg Nurs* 13:83, 1981

Plank N: Multiple sclerosis: An update and review. *J Neurosurg Nurs* 11:44, 1979

Rasmussen D: Amyotrophic lateral sclerosis. *Am J Nurs* 80:2050, 1980

Swift N: Why the MS patient needs your help. *Nursing* 9:57, Sept 1979

Chapter 11

Bowens B: Carpal tunnel syndrome: *J Neurosurg Nurs* 13:129, 1981

Hrovath M: Myasthenia gravis: A nursing approach. *J Neurosurg Nurs* 14:7, 1982

Mills N, Plasterer H H: Guillain-Barré syndrome: A framework for nursing care. *Nurs Clin North Am* 15:257, 1980

Morris J: Thymectomy: A recommended procedure for myasthenia gravis. *J Neurosurg Nurs* 13:226, 1981

Ostrow L: New hope for patients with trigeminal neuralgia. *Am J Nurs* 76:1301, 1976

Tikkanen P: Landry-Guillain-Barré-Strohl syndrome. *J Neurosurg Nurs* 14:74, 1982

Chapter 12

Blount M, Kinney A: What to remember about EEG. *Nursing,* p 36, Aug 1974

Bubb D: Neurodiagnostic studies: Pre- and post-procedure care. *RN* 44:64, Nov 1981

Bubb D: Teaching patients about ultrasound and CAT brain scans. *RN* 44:64, Dec 1981

Bubb D: Helping your patient through two painful tests. *RN* 45:64, Jan 1982

Bubb D: Neurodiagnostic studies: Pre- and post-procedure care. *RN* 45:64, Feb 1982

Donahoe J, Blount M, Kinney A: Cerebral circulation and cerebral angiography. *Nurs Clin North Am* 9:623, 1974

Lamb S: The nurse's changing role in water-soluble myelography. *J Neurosurg Nurs* 78:189, 1978

Lyons M, Wilson D: Regional cerebral blood flow – A newer non-invasive neurodiagnostic test. *J Neurosurg Nurs* 13:286, 1981

Mandrillo M: Brain scanning. *Nurs Clin North Am* 9:633, 1974

Ross A, et al: Neuromuscular diagnostic procedures. *Nurs Clin North Am* 14:107, 1979

INDEX

A

Abdominal reflex, 59
Abducens nerve, 16, 45-46
Absence (petit mal) seizures, 99-100
Acetylcholine, 5, 21
Achilles reflex, 58, *59**
Acoustic nerve, 16, 48
Acoustic neuroma, 147
Acquired epilepsy, 96-97
Action potential (neurons), 4
Adrenal, *20*, 22
Adrenergic fibers, 21
Adrenocorticotropin (ACTH), 208-209
Agnosia, 42
Airway
 head injury, 132
 intracranial pressure management, 73
 patient management, 78, 79
Alcohol use, 36, 97
Alexia, 43
Allergies, 35
Alopecia, 151
Amantadine, 167, 170, 208-209
Ambu bag, 79
Ambulation, 79. *See also* Mobility
Aminocaproic acid, 120, 208-209
Aminophylline, 120
Amitriptyline, 172
Amyotrophic lateral sclerosis, 171-174
Aneurysms. *See* Cerebral aneurysms
Angiography (cerebral), 201-202
Ankle clonus, 58
Anosmia, 43
Anterior cerebral artery, *12*
 occlusion, 114
Anterior communicating artery, *12*
Anterior cord syndrome, 135
Anterior funiculi, 13
Anterior inferior cerebellar artery, occlusion, 115
Anterior spinothalamic tract, 14
Anticholinergic drugs, *167*, 170
Anticholinesterase drugs, 180
Anticoagulants, 116
Anticonvulsant drugs, 73, 103, *104*
Antihistaminic drugs, *167*, 170
Antihypertensive drugs, 120
Aphasia, 42-43, 89, 151
Apneustic breathing, 67
Appetite, 33, 84
Aqueduct of Sylvius, *9*, 11
Arachnoid membrane, 7
Arachnoid villi, 11
Areflexic (atonic) bladder, 87
Arm strength, 54
Arousal, 64
Arrhythmias, 68
Arteriovenous malformations (AVMs), 122-123
Aspirin, 80
Assessment, 39-62
 amyotrophic lateral sclerosis, 173-174
 aneurysms, 120-122
 arteriovenous malformations, 123
 brain tumor, 148-152
 cerebellar function, 50
 cerebral function, 41-43
 cognitive functions, 40-41
 consciousness, 64-69
 cranial nerve functions, 43-50
 general observations in, 40
 Guillain-Barré syndrome, 184
 head injury, 132-133
 motor function, 52-55

---

*Italic page numbers refer to illustrations.

multiple sclerosis, 162-165
myasthenia gravis, 180-181
Parkinson's disease, 168-171
rationale for, 40
reflex evaluation, 56-60
seizures, 101-105
sensory evaluation, 51-52
spinal cord injury, 137-138, 140
spinal cord tumors, 155-156
stroke, 116-117
Associative auditory cortex, *8*
Astereognosis, 42
Astrocytes, 2
Astrocytoma, 146, 153
Ataxia, 53, 103, *111*, 163
Ataxic breathing, 68
Atelectasis, 79
Atherosclerotic changes, 110, 111
Athetosis, 53
Atonic (areflexic) bladder, 87, 140
Atonic seizures, 100
Atrophy, 53
Atropine, 181, 208-209
Auditory agnosia, 42
Auditory cortex, 8
Auditory disturbances, 32
Auditory stimulus, 64
Autonomic hyperreflexia, 139
Autonomic nervous system, 6, 21, *22*, *23*
Axons, 2, *3*, 4, 5

B

Babinski reflex, 59, *60*, 69, 132
Back pain, 153
Baclofen, 163, 164, 208-209
Balance, 48, 50
Barbiturate coma, 73
Basal ganglia, 9
Basilar artery, *12*
Benign tumors, 146, 152
Benztropine, *167*
Berry aneurysms, 118

Bethanechol, 164, 208-209
Biceps reflex, *56*, 57
Biochemical disorders causing seizures, 97
Biperiden, *167*
Bipolar neurons, 4
Bladder, *20, 22, 23*, 87. *See also entries under* Urinary
Bladder control. *See* Incontinence
Blood
  brain tumor chemotherapy, 151
  cerebral circulation, 11-12
Blood-brain barrier, 2, 12
Blood pressure. *See also* Hypertension; Hypotension
  autonomic nervous responses, *22*
  intracranial pressure, 68, 70, 71
Body alignment. *See* Positioning
Body temperature
  intracranial pressure, 71, 73
  level of consciousness, 68
  multiple sclerosis, 162
Bone marrow depression, 151, 152
Bowel elimination, 85-86
  amyotrophic lateral sclerosis, 174
  multiple sclerosis, 164
  Parkinson's disease, 168-169
  patient history, 33
  spinal cord injury, *136-137*
Bowel sounds, 85, 149, 150
Bowel training, 86
Brachial plexus, 19
Brachioradialis (supinator) reflex, 58
Bradycardia, 68, 132
Brain
  arteriovenous malformations, 122
  assessment, 41-43

blood-brain barrier, 12
brain stem, 10
cerebellar function assessment, 50
cerebellum, 10
cerebral circulation, 11-12
cerebrum, 7-8
consciousness and, 64
cranium and, 6
intracranial pressure, 70
meninges, 7
specialized systems of, 10
stroke and, 110-111, 113-115
venous drainage of, 12
ventricular system, 11
Brain lesion, 97-98
Brain scan, 196-197
Brain stem, 10
Brain tumors
chemotherapy for, 151
classification, 145-148
diagnosis, 148
nursing assessment in, 148-152
pathophysiology, 144-145
radiation therapy for, 152
signs and symptoms, 145
Broca's area, 7, 8
Bronchi, 22, 23
Brown-Sequard syndrome, 135, 154
Bureau of Vocational Rehabilitation, 165

C

Carbamazepine, *104*, 208-209
Carbidopa, 167, 208-209
Carbon dioxide, 70
Cardiac monitoring, 80
Carotid arteries, 11, *111*, 112
Carotid artery occlusion, 114
Carpal tunnel syndrome, 185-187
Catechol O-methyltransferase (COMT), 5
Catheterization, 87, 88
intracranial pressure and, 73
multiple sclerosis, 164
spinal cord injury, 140
CAT scan. *See* Computed tomography
Cauda equina, 17
Cavernous sinus, 12
Cells, nervous system, 2-4
Central cord syndrome, 135
Central nervous system, 5. *See also* Brain; Spinal cord
bony structures, 6
brain anatomy, 7-12
cerebrum, 7-8
meningeal spaces, 7
trauma, 127-142. *See also* Head trauma, Spinal cord injury
tumors. *See* Brain tumors; Spinal cord tumors
Central neurogenic hyperventilation, 67
Central sulcus, 8
Cerebellar artery occlusion, 114, 115
Cerebellum, 8, 9, 10, 50
Cerebral aneurysms
diagnosis, 119
etiology, 118-119
medical management, 120
nursing assessment and management, 120-122
progression and complications in, 119-120
signs and symptoms, 119
stroke and, 113
Cerebral angiography, 201-202
Cerebral artery occlusion, 113-114
Cerebral blood flow, 70
diagnostic procedure for, 197-198
patient management, 80
stroke and, 110
Cerebral contusion, 130
Cerebral edema, 83, 128, 144
Cerebral function, 41-43
Cerebral hematoma, 129

Cerebral hemorrhage, 129
Cerebral metabolism, 64
Cerebral tissue damage, 128
Cerebral vasospasm, 119-120
Cerebrospinal fluid, 11
   brain tumor and, 145, 150
   Guillain-Barré syndrome, 184
   head injury, 132
   intracranial pressure, 70, 73
   lumbar puncture, 198-199
   multiple sclerosis, 161
   normal values, *199*
   spinal cord tumors, 154
Cerebrovascular accident. *See* Stroke
Cerebrovascular diseases, 109-125
   arteriovenous malformations, 122-123
   cerebral aneurysms, 118-122
   stroke, 110-118. *See also* Stroke
Cerebrum, 7-8, 128
Cervical nerves, 17, 19
Cervical plexus, 19
Cervical spine injury, 136
Cervical vertebrae, 6
Chaddock reflex, 59
Charcot-Marie-Tooth disease, 203
Chemotherapy, 151, 155
Cheyne-Stokes respiration, 67
Childhood-onset brain tumors, 146
Chloride ions, 4
Chlorphenoxamine, *167*
Cholesterol levels, 110
Cholinergic crisis, 181-182
Cholinergic fibers, 21
Cholinesterase, 5
Chorea, 53
Choroid plexus, 11
Cigarette smoking. *See* Tobacco
Cimetidine, 155, 208-209
Circle of Willis, 11, *12*, 110, 118, 119

Circulatory system, 79-80
Clonazepam, *104*
Cluster breathing, 67
Coccygeal nerves, 17
Coccygeal vertebrae, 6
Cognition, 40-41, 64
Collagen disease, 110
Coma. *See also* Consciousness
   body temperature, 68
   causes, 64
   defined, 65
   eye care in, 93
   seizure and, 98
   stroke and, 113
Communication. *See also* Aphasia; Language; Speech; Writing disorders
   amyotrophic lateral sclerosis, 173
   brain tumor surgery, 151
   patient management, 88-89
   Parkinson's disease, 169
Complex partial seizures, 98
Computed tomography (CT or CAT scan), 194-196
   head injury, 131
   multiple sclerosis, 162
   spinal cord tumor, 155
Concussion, 129-130
Conductivity, 2
Confusion, *111*
Consciousness, 64-69
   intracranial pressure and, 71
   nutrition and, 84
   See also Coma
Constipation, 86, 140. *See also* Bowel elimination
Contrecoup lesion, 128
Conus medullaris, 13
Convulsions, 31. *See also* Seizures
Corneal reflex, *47*, 82-83, 150
Corpus callosum, *9*
Corticoreticulospinal tract, 14
Corticorubrospinal tract, 14
Corticospinal tract, 14, 56

Corticosteroids, 73, 155, 180-181. *See also* Steroids
Coughing, 72, 78, 79, 165, 169
Coup lesions, 128
Cranial nerves, 14-17, 21
   acoustic neuroma, 147
   amyotrophic lateral sclerosis, 171
   assessment of, 43-50
   brain stem and, 10
   brain tumor surgery, 151
   disturbed function, 32-33
   Guillain-Barré syndrome, 183, 184
   head injury, 129
Craniotomy, 83
Cranium, 6
Credé method, 87, *137*, 164
Cremasteric reflex, 59
CT scan. *See* Computed tomography
Cycrimine, *167*

D

Dantrolene, 140, 163, 172, 210-211
Decerebrate posturing, 69
Decorticate posturing, 69
Decussation, 14, *15*
Deep tendon reflexes, 56-58, 132
Degenerative diseases
   amyotrophic lateral sclerosis, 171-174
   multiple sclerosis, 160-165
   Parkinson's disease, 165-171
Delirium, 65
Dendrites, 3, 4, 5
Deoxyribonucleic acid (DNA) 3
Depolarization, 4, 5
Dermatomes, *18*
Dexamethasone, 116, 120, 139, 210-211
Diabetes insipidus, 83, 149-150
Diabetes mellitus, 110
Diagnostic procedures
   brain scan, 196-197
   cerebral angiography, 201-202
   computed tomography, 194-196
   echoencephalography, 196
   electroencephalogram, 193-194
   electromyography (EMG), 203
   lumbar puncture, 198-199
   myelography, 199-201
   nerve conduction studies, 203-204
   noninvasive regional cerebral blood flow, 197-198
   radiology, 192-193
Diarrhea, 85, 86
Diazepam, *104*, 140, 163, 172, 210-211
Diencephalon, 8, 10
Dietitian, 84, 173
Digestive system, *20, 22, 23*
Diphenhydramine, *167*
Diplopia, 90, 103, 163, 180
Discriminatory sensation, 51-52
Discs, intervertebral, 6
Diuretics, 73
Dopamine, 5, *167*
Dorsal root ganglia, 18, *19*
Dorsiflexion of foot, 55
Drugs, 36
Drug therapy. *See* Pharmacology; *entries under names of specific drugs*
Dural sinuses, 12
Dura mater, 7
Dysarthria. *See* Speech
Dysphagia. *See* Swallowing disorders

E

Ears, 34. *See also* Hearing
Ecchymosis, 83
Echoencephalography, 196
Edema, 79, 93
Edrophonium (Tensilon) test, 179

Education. *See* Patient education
Educational history, 35
Elbow strength, 54
Electroencephalogram (EEG), 101, 193-194
Electromyography (EMG), 180, 203
Elimination. *See* Bowel elimination; Incontinence
Embolic stroke, 112-113
Emotional needs
  amyotrophic lateral sclerosis, 174
  aneurysms, 122
  assessment, 40
  brain tumor surgery, 151
  history, 29, 33
  multiple sclerosis, 162-163, 164
  Parkinson's disease, 169-170
  patient management, 90-91
Encephalitis, 165
Endoplasmic reticulum, 3
Endotracheal tube, 79
Enemas, 86
Enzymes, neurotransmitter inactivation, 5
Ependymal cells, 2
Ependymomas, 153
Epidural hematoma, 130
Epidural space, 7
Epilepsy, 96, 99, 100. *See also* Seizures
Epithalamus, 8, *9*
Esophagostomy, 173
Esophagus, *20, 23*
Ethmoid bone, *6*
Ethosuximide, *104*
Excitatory neurotransmitters, 5
Exercise
  amyotrophic lateral sclerosis, 174
  multiple sclerosis, 163
  patient management, 81
  seizures and, 105

spinal cord injury, 140
Expressive aphasia, 43, 89
Extinction phenomenon, 52
Extradural tumors, 153
Extramedullary tumors, 153, 155
Extrapyramidal tract, *15*
Extravertebral tumors, 153
Eyelids, 46
Eyes
  assessment, 44-46
  autonomic nervous responses, *22*
  care, 82-83
  consciousness, 65-67
  head injury, 132
  history, 34
  multiple sclerosis, 163
  myasthenia gravis, 178
  parasympathetic control, *23*
  Parkinson's disease, 171
  sympathetic control, *20*

F

Face, 33, 46-47
Facial nerve, 16, 47-48
Family, 90-91
  amyotrophic lateral sclerosis, 173, 174
  aneurysms, 121
  brain tumor patients, 151, 152
  Parkinson's disease, 169-170
  stroke patients, 118
Family history, 36
Feeding, 85
Fever, 149
Filum terminale, 13
Finger strength, 55
Fluid restriction, 121
Fluid volume, 83
Focal seizures, 98
Foot, 55, 58, 59
Foramen of Monro, *9*, 11
Fornix, *9*
Fourth ventricle, *9*
Frontal bone, *6*
Frontal lobe, 7, *8*

G

Gait, 28, 52-53, 163
Gamma-aminobutyric acid, 5
Ganglia, sympathetic nervous system, 20
Gas exchange, 78
Gastrointestinal tract, 33, 35
Gastrostomy tube, 84, 85, 173
Generalized seizures, 98-100
Genitourinary system, 20, 23, 35
Glasgow coma scale (GCS), 65, 66, 132
Glaucoma, 171
Glossopharyngeal nerve, 16, 48-49
Glycine, 5
Golgi apparatus, 3
Gordon reflex, 60
Grand mal seizures, 98, 99
Graphesthesia, 52
Grasp reflex, 69
Great longitudinal fissure, 7
Grieving process, 90
Grip strength, 55
Guillain-Barré syndrome, 182-185, 203
  communication impairment, 89
  patient management, 79

H

Hallucination, 65
Handedness, 29, 115
Headache
  aneurysms, 119, 121
  intracranial pressure, 72
  patient history, 30
  transient ischemic attacks, 111
Head trauma, 128-133
  history, 33-34
Hearing, 48
Heart
  autonomic nervous responses, 22
  Guillain-Barré syndrome, 184
  head injury, 132
  parasympathetic control, 23
  patient history, 34
  patient management, 79-80
  stroke and, 110, 112
  sympathetic control, 20
Hemangioblastoma, 147
Hematoma, 129, 130-131
Hemianopsia, 90, 115
Hemiparesis, 52, 71
Hemiplegia, 71, 115
Hemorrhage, 129, 131, 151
Hemorrhagic stroke, 113
Heparin, 80, 112, 184, 210-211
Hip motion, 55
History. See Patient history
Hydrocephalus, 70, 145, 150
Hygiene, 82-83, 169
Hypercapnia, 70, 72, 79, 128
Hypertension. See also Blood pressure; Hypotension
  aneurysms, 120
  head injury, 132
  spinal cord injury, 139
  stroke and, 110, 113
Hyperventilation, 67, 73
Hypoglossal nerve, 17, 50
Hypotension, 80. See also Blood pressure; Hypertension
  head injury, 132
  Parkinson's disease, 169
  spinal cord injury, 139
Hypothalamus, 9, 68
Hypothermia. See Body temperature
Hypothermia blanket, 82
Hypovolemic shock, 150
Hypoxemia, 72

I

Idiopathic epilepsy, 96
Impotence, 154, 164
Impulse conduction, 4-5
Incontinence
  multiple sclerosis, 164
  Parkinson's disease, 169
  patient management, 82, 86-88

spinal cord injury, 140
spinal cord tumors, 154, 156
Infection
　body temperature, 68
　brain tumor chemotherapy, 151
　catheters, 87, 88
　multiple sclerosis, 164
　patient management, 81
　spinal cord injury, 140
Inferior longitudinal sinus, 12
Inhibitory neurotransmitters, 5
Injury, 88. *See also* Head trauma; Spinal cord injury
Internal capsule, *15*
Internal carotid artery, *12*
　occlusion, 115
International Classification of Epileptic Seizures, 97
Internuncial neuron, *19*
Interthalamic adhesion, *9*
Intervertebral discs, 6
Intestines, *20, 23*
Intracerebral hemotoma, 130-131
Intracranial pressure, 69-74
　alterations in, 70
　aneurysms and, 121
　brain tumors and, 149, 150
　coughing and, 78
　dynamics, 69-70
　enemas and, 86
　factors affecting, 72-73
　head injury and, 128, 129
　management of increases in, 73-74
　pulse and, 68
　signs and symptoms of increased, 71-72
Intradural tumors, 153
Intramedullary tumors, 153
Intravenous feedings, 85
Irritability, 2
Ischemia, 120, 129
Isometric exercise, 72-73
Isoproterenol, 120

J

"Jacksonian march," 98
Judgment, 41

K

Kanamycin, 120
Kidney, *20, 23*
Knee motion, 55, 58
Knowledge deficit, 91

L

Laboratory studies, 138, *199*
Lacrimal bone, *6*
Lacrimal gland, *20, 23*
Language, 42-43. *See also* Speech
Larynx, *20, 23*
Lateral ventricle, *9*
Laxatives, 86, 121
L-Dopa (levodopa), 167, 170, 208-209, 210-211
Libido, 33
Liver, *20, 22, 23*
Lower motor neuron, *15*
Lumbar nerves, 17, *19*
Lumbar plexus, 19
Lumbar puncture (spinal tap), 131, 154, 184, 198-199
Lumbar spine injury, 137
Lumbar vertebrae, 6
Lungs, *20, 23*, 34. *See also* Respiration

M

Maalox, 155
Mandible, *6*
Mannitol, 116, 210-211
Masseter muscle, 47
Maxilla, *6*
Median nerve, 185, 186, 187
Medic Alert bracelets, 105
Medulla, *9*, 10, *20*
Memory, 41
Meninges, 7
Meningiomas, 147, 152, 153
Menstruation, 35, 105

237

Mental status. *See* Emotional needs
Microglia, 2
Midbrain, 9, 10, *20*
Middle cerebral artery occlusion, 113-114
Mitochondria, 3
Mobility, 79
  amyotrophic lateral sclerosis, 174
  Parkinson's disease, 168, 169
  patient management, 80-81
Monoamine oxidase (MAO), 5
Monro-Kellie hypothesis, 69-70
Motor area, *8*, *15*
Motor association area, 7
Motor dysfunction
  intracranial pressure and, 71
  multiple sclerosis, 163, 164-165
  myasthenia gravis, 178-179
  Parkinson's disease, 168
  spinal cord tumors, 153, 155
Motor end plate, *3*
Motor function, 28, 52-55, 68-69
Motor integration, 42
Motor neuron, *3*, *19*
Motor tracts, 14
Mouth, 34, 82, 151
Movement disorders, 32, 52-53
Mucous membranes, *20*, *23*
Multiple sclerosis, 160-165
Multipolar neurons, 4
Muscle, *3*, *19*, 52-55, 56
Myasthenia gravis, 79, 84, 178-182
Myasthenic crisis, 181-182
Myelin sheath, 2, *3*, 4
Myelography, 138, 154, 199-201
Myoclonic seizures, 100

N

Nail care, 83
Nasogastric tubes, 84, 85, 173
National Multiple Sclerosis Society, 165

Nausea/vomiting, *111*
Neck pain, 153
Neostigmine, 172, 180, 210-211
Neostigmine (Prostigmin) test, 180
Nerve conduction studies, 203-204
Nervous system, anatomy and physiology, 1-25
Neurinomas, 153
Neuroglia cells, 1
Neurolemma, 4
Neurologic assessment. *See* Assessment
Neuromuscular diseases
  Carpal tunnel syndrome, 185-187
  Guillain-Barré syndrome, 182-185
  myasthenia gravis, 178-182
Neurons, 2-4
Neurotransmitters, 5
Nissl bodies, 3, 4
Node of Ranvier, *3*, 4
Norepinephrine, 5, 21
Nose, 34
Number identification, 52
Nursing assessment. *See* Assessment
Nutrition
  amyotrophic lateral sclerosis, 173
  brain tumor, 151, 152
  constipation and, 86
  neuronal, 2
  Parkinson's disease, 168
  patient management, 83-85
Nystagmus, 103

O

Obesity, 110
Occipital bone, 6
Occiptal lobe, *8*
Occupational history, 35
Occupational therapy, 169
Ocular myasthenia, 179
Oculomotor nerve, 16, 45-46, 71

Olfactory disturbances, 32-33
Olfactory nerve, 15, 43
Oligoclonal bands, 161
Oligodendroglia, 2
Oligodendroglioma, 146
Ophthalmoscopic examination, 44-45. *See also* Eyes
Oppenheim reflex, 60
Optic chiasm, *9*
Optic discs, 44, 45
Optic nerve, 16, 44-45
Oral contraceptives, 110
Orphenadrine, *167*
Orthopedic history, 35
Orthostatic hypotension, 80, 139, 169. *See also* Blood pressure; hypotension
Oxygen therapy, 78, 173

P

Pain
   amyotrophic lateral sclerosis, 174
   assessment, *46*
   patient history, 30
   patient management, 88
   sensitivity, 51, 64
   spinal cord tumors, 153, 156
   thalamus and, 8
Pancreas, *20, 23*
Papilledema, 45, 72, 154
Paralysis, 80. *See also* Hemiplegia; Paraplegia; Quadriplegia
   Guillain-Barré syndrome, 183
   seizure and, 98
   spinal cord injury, 134, 136-137
Paraplegia, *136-137*
Parasympathetic nervous system, 21-23
Parenteral hyperalimentation, 85
Paresthesia, *111*
Parietal bones, 6
Parietal lobe, 7, *8*

Parkinsonian gait, 53
Parkinson's disease, 81, 165-166, *167*, 168-171
Parotid gland, *20, 23*
Partial seizures, 97-98
Patellar reflex, 58
Patient education, 91
   amyotrophic lateral sclerosis, 173
   brain tumor, 148-149, 152
   carpal tunnel syndrome, 187
   multiple sclerosis, 162-163
   Parkinson's disease, 170
   seizures, 103, 105
   spinal cord injury, 156
   stroke patients, 117-118
Patient history, 28-36
   educational history, 35
   family history, 36
   interview, 29-36
   observations during, 28-29
   occupational history, 35
   past history, 34
   personal habits, 34
   personality inventory, 35
   seizures, 101-102
   spinal cord injury, 138
   symptoms and, 29-34
   systems review, 34-35
Patient management, 77-93
   amyotrophic lateral sclerosis, 172-173
   aneurysms, 120-122
   arteriovenous malformations, 123
   carpal tunnel syndrome, 186-187
   Guilllain-Barré syndrome, 184, 185
   head injury, 131-132
   multiple sclerosis, 162
   myasthenia gravis, 182
   Parkinson's disease, 166-167
   seizures, 99, 102
   spinal cord injury, 138-139, 140

spinal cord tumors, 155-156
Periocular edema, 83
Peripheral nerve damage, 87
Peripheral nervous system
   autonomic nervous system, 21-23
   cranial nerves, 14-17
   spinal nerves, 17-21
Peristalsis, 85
Personality, 33, 35
Petit mal (absence) seizures, 99-100
Phagocytosis, 2
Phalen's sign, 186
Pharmacology
   amyotrophic lateral sclerosis, 172
   aneurysms, 120, 121
   anticonvulsant therapy, 103
   brain tumor chemotherapy, 151
   Guillain-Barré syndrome, 184
   intracranial pressure and, 73
   listings of drugs, 208-211
   multiple sclerosis, 163, 164
   myasthenia gravis, 180-181
   Parkinson's disease, 165, 166-167, 170
   spinal cord injury, 139, 140
   spinal cord tumors, 155
   stroke, 116
Phenobarbital, *104*
Phenothiazines, 165
Phenytoin, 104
Phrenic nerve, 19
Physical therapy, 172, 174. *See also* Exercise
Pia mater, 7
Pin and tong sites, 81
Pituitary, 9, 10, 145
Pituitary tumors, 147
Plantar flexion of foot, 55
Plantar reflex, 59
Plasmapheresis, 181
Plexuses, 19

Point discrimination tests, 52
Pons, 9, 10
Positioning, 79
   intracranial pressure and, 73
   patient management, 80-81
Posterior cerebral artery, *12*
   occlusion, 114
Posterior columns, 14
Posterior communicating artery, *12*
Posterior funiculi, 13
Posterior inferior cerebellar artery occlusion, 114
Postsynaptic membrane, 5
Post-traumatic epilepsy 97
Posture, 28
Posturing, decerebrate and decorticate, 69
Potassium ions, 4
Prednisone, 104, 180-181, 210-211
Pregnancy, 105, 164
Premotor area, 8, *15*
Premotor cortex, 7
Presenting complaint, 29
Pressure sensitivity, 51
Presynaptic terminal, 5
Primary auditory cortex, *8*
Primary motor area, 7
Primary sensory cortex, 7
Primidone, 104
Principal motor area, *8*
Principal sensory areas, *8*
Principal visual cortex, *8*
Procyclidine, *167*
Propantheline bromide, 172
Prostigmin (neostigmine) test, 180
Ptosis, 46, 180
Pulmonary toilet, 78
Pulse, 68, 71
Pupils, 46, 65-67, 71. *See also* Eyes
Pyramidal tract, *15*
Pyramidal tract disease, 59
Pyridostigmine, 180, 210-211

Q

Quadriplegia, *136*, *137*
Queckenstedt's sign, 154

R

Radiation therapy, 152, 155
Radicular pain, 153
Radioactive isotopes, 196-198
Radiology
 head injury, 131
 myelography, 199-201
 spinal cord injury, 138
 spinal cord tumor, 154
Rapid eye movement sleep, 73
Rauwolfia alkaloids, 165
Reading disorders, 43
Receptive aphasia, 42-43, 89
Receptor, *19*
Rectum, *20*, *23*
Reflex arc, *19*, 21
Reflexes
 assessment, *47*, 56-60
 coma, 65
 consciousness, 69
 deep tendon reflexes, 56-58
 head injury, 133
 nerves and, 19, 21
 pathologic, 59, *60*
Rehabilitation
 head injury, 133
 patient management, 91
 spinal cord injury, 141
Repolarization, 4
Reproductive system, 35
Reserpine, 120, 165
Respiration
 amyotrophic lateral sclerosis, 173
 autonomic nervous responses, *22*
 brain tumor, 149
 consciousness, 67-68
 Guillain-Barré syndrome, 184, 185
 head injury, 132
 intracranial pressure and, 71
 multiple sclerosis, 164-165
 myasthenia gravis, 179
 Parkinson's disease, 169
 patient management, 78-79
 spinal cord injury, *136-137*, 139
 spinal cord tumors, 155
Resting membrane potential, 4
Restraints, 88
Reticular activating system, 10
Reticular formation, 10
Reuptake mechanism, 5
Rib cage, 134
Ribonucleic acid (RNA), 3
Rinne test, 48
Romberg test, 50, 103

S

Sacral nerves, 17, 19
Sacral plexus, 19
Sacral spine injury, 137
Sacral vertebrae, 6
Safety, 88, *102*, 168
Saltatory conduction, 4
Schwann cell, *3*, 4
Scissors gait, 52
Secondary generalized seizures, 98
Sedatives, 120
Seizures, 95-107. *See also* Epilepsy
 aneurysms, 121
 anticonvulsant drugs, 104
 brain tumors, 145, 150
 classification, 97-100
 defined, 96
 diagnosis, 100-101
 etiology, 96-97
 nursing assessment, 101-105
 nursing responsibilities, *99*
 safety and, 88, *102*
Self-care deficits, 82-83
Sensation disorders, 32
Sensory ability, 7
Sensory association areas, 7, *8*
Sensory function
 assessment, 42, 51-52

consciousness, 68
Guillain-Barré syndrome, 183
intracranial pressure and, 71
multiple sclerosis, 163
patient management, 89-90
spinal cord tumors, 154, 155
Sensory neuron, *19*
Sensory tract, 14
Serotonin, 5
Sexuality, 154, 164
Shoulder strength, 54
Simple partial seizures, 98
Skin
   amyotrophic lateral sclerosis, 174
   autonomic nervous responses, *22*
   brain tumor radiation therapy, 152
   dermatomes, *18*
   history, 35
   incontinence, 87
   multiple sclerosis, 165
   Parkinson's disease, 169
   patient management, 81-82
   spinal cord tumors, 156
   superficial reflexes, 58-59
   traction patients, 81
Skull, 6, 128
Skull fracture, 128, 129, 131
Skull X-ray, 131, 192
Sleep, 73
Sleep disorders, 33
Slings, 80
Smoking. *See* Tobacco
Sneezing, 72
Social workers, 165
Sodium ions, 4, 5
Soma, 2, *3*, 5
Somatic awareness, 7
Spastic hemiparesis, 52
Spasticity, 81, 140, 163. *See also* Seizures
Spatial agnosia, 42
Spatial orientation, 7
Speech, 7
   amyotrophic lateral sclerosis, 173
   hemiplegia, *115*
   history, 33
   multiple sclerosis, 164
   myasthenia gravis, 178
   Parkinson's disease, 169
   transient ischemic attacks, *111*
Speech therapists and therapy, 84, 89, 164, 173
Sphenoid bone, *6*
Sphincter control, 156
Spinal accessory nerve, 16, *49*, 50
Spinal cord, *19*
   amyotrophic lateral sclerosis, 171
   anatomy, *13*, 14
   vertebrae, 6
Spinal cord injury
   assessment, 137-138
   functional loss and expectations following, 135, *136-137*
   medical management, 138-139
   nursing assessment, 140
   problems and complications, 139-140
   rehabilitation, 141
   signs and symptoms, 134-135
   urinary elimination, 87
Spinal cord tumors
   classification of, 153
   diagnosis of, 154-155
   medical management in, 155
   nursing care in, 155-156
   pathophysiology of, 152
   signs and symptoms of, 153-154
Spinal nerves, *17*, 18-21
Spinal shock, 134
Spinal tap. *See* Lumbar puncture

Spinocerebellar tracts, 14
Spinothalamic tracts, 14
Splints, 80
Status epilepticus, 96, 99, 100.
  See also Seizures
Steppage gait, 53
Stereognostic function, 52
Sternocleidomastoid muscle, 49
Steroids, 139, 184
Stomach, *20, 23*
Stomatitis, 151
Stool softeners, 86, 121
Striated muscle, *3*
Stroke
  classification, 111-113
  completed, 112
  defined, 110
  diagnosis, 115-116
  discharge planning assessment, 117-118
  epidemiology, 110
  hemiplegia, 115
  medical management, 116
  nursing assessment and management, 116-117
  pathophysiology, 110-111
  patient management, 79, 80
  predisposing factors, 110
  prognosis, 113
  symptoms, 113-115
Stroke-in-evolution, 112, 116
Subarachnoid hemorrhage, 131
Subarachnoid space, 7
Subdural hematoma, 130
Subdural space, 7
Sublingual gland, *20, 23*
Submaxillary gland, *20, 23*
Subthalamus, *9*
Suctioning, 78, 79
Superior longitudinal sinus, 12
Supinator (brachioradialis) reflex, *58*
Suppositories, rectal, 86
Surgery
  aneurysms, 120
  brain tumor, 149-151, 152
  spinal cord injury, 139, 140
  spinal cord tumor, 155
  stroke, 112, 116
Sutures, 6
Swallowing disorders, 84
  amyotrophic lateral sclerosis, 173
  history, 33
  myasthenia gravis, 178, 180
Sympathetic nervous system, *20*, 21
Synapse, 5
Synaptic cleft, 5

T

Tachycardia, 68, 132
Tactile sensation, 42, 51, 90
Taste, 32-33, 47-48
Temperature. *See* Body temperature
Temperature sensitivity, 51
Temporal bones, 6
Temporal lobe, *8*
Temporal lobe seizures, 98
Temporal muscle, 47
Tensilon (edrophonium) test, 179
Tentorium cerebelli, 7
Texture discrimination, 52
Thalamus, 8, *9*
Third ventricle, *9*
Thirst, 33
Thoracic nerves, 17, 19
Thoracic spine injury, 136-137
Thoracic vertebrae, 6
Throat. *See* Mouth
Thrombophlebitis, 79-80, 121, 139
Thrombotic stroke, 111-112, 113
Thrombus, 110, 111
Thymectomy, 181
Tics, 53
Tinel's sign, 186
Tinnitus, 48
Tobacco, 36, 110

Todd's paralysis, 98
Tonic-clonic (grand mal) seizures, *99*
Tooth care, 82
Toxins, 97, 103
Trachea, *20, 23*
Tracheostomy, 184
    patient management, 79
    speech impairment and, 88, 89
Traction, 81
Transient ischemic attacks (TIA), *111*, 112
Trapezius muscle, 49, 50
Trauma. *See also* Head trauma; Spinal cord injury
    seizures and, 97
    stroke and, 113
Tremors, 53
Trendelenburg's position, 73
Triceps reflex, *57*
Trigeminal nerve, 16, *46, 47*
Trihexyphenidyl, *167*, 172
Trimethadione, *104*
Trochlear nerve, 16, 45-46
Tumors. *See* Brain tumors; Spinal cord tumors
Two-point discrimination tests, 51

U

Unconsciousness, 88. *See also* Coma
Unipolar neurons, 4
Upper motor neuron disease, 56
Urea, 210-211
Urinary bladder training, 87
Urinary elimination, *136-137*
Urinary output, 93
Urinary problems, 33
Urine testing, 87, 149-150

V

Vagus nerve, 16, 48-49, 183
Valproic acid, *104*
Valsalva's maneuver, 72, 86, 121, 153
Vascular system, 45
Vasodilating drugs, 73
Vasopressin, 150, 210-211
Vasospasms, 119-120
Venous drainage, 12
Ventilators, 79
Ventral roots, *19*
Ventricular system, 11
Vertebrae, 6, 133
Vertebral arteries, 11, *12*
Vertebrobasilar system, *111*,112
Vertigo, 31, 48, *111*
Vestibulospinal tract, 14
Vibration sensitivity, 51
Visceral disorders, 33
Visual agnosia, 42
Visual association areas, 8
Visual cortex, *8*
Visual defects, 32, 89-90, *111*
Visual evoked response, 162
Vital signs
    head injury, 132
    intracranial pressure and, 71
    spinal cord tumors, 155
Vomiting, 33, 72

W

Warfarin, 184
Wrist
    carpal tunnel syndrome, 185
    strength, 54
Writing, 169
Writing disorders, 43

X

X-ray. *See* Radiology